Herbal Strategies Against Viruses

Harnessing the Power of Botanicals in Viral Infections

Richard Fieldstone

Table of Contents

INTRODUCTION

Provides a thorough investigation of plants' practical impact in preventing viral infections. Written by Richard Fieldstone, this book is an essential and current resource in light of the problems that viral outbreaks pose to the world.

Traditional herbal medicines have gained popularity again as an adjuvant or substitute therapy for antiviral drugs. There is an increasing need to investigate new therapeutic approaches since viruses are changing and resistant to current treatments. This book explores the vast repertoire of botanicals, utilizing contemporary scientific research and age-old knowledge to clarify their effectiveness against various viral infections.

The foundation is laid in the first few chapters, which cover the fundamentals of herbal therapy, the mechanisms behind viral infections, and the justification for including botanicals in conventional antiviral treatments. Readers are taken on a trip that offers insights into the chemical connections between viral targets and bioactive molecules in plants, bridging the gap between traditional wisdom and modern scientific understanding.

The book identifies attractive candidates for more research and clinical validation by comprehensively evaluating botanicals with known antiviral activities. Every plant profile, including lesser-known species with antiviral solid activity and well-known plants like elderberry and echinacea, is carefully recorded with its historical applications, phytochemical components, and evidence-based recommendations in viral infections.
The book examines botanicals' immunomodulatory, anti-inflammatory, and tissue-protective qualities in addition

to their direct antiviral activities, highlighting their comprehensive strategy for treating viral illnesses. In addition, it covers issues like quality assurance, safety, and regulations, guaranteeing a fair viewpoint on incorporating herbal medicine into clinical practice.

For researchers, medical experts, and herbal lovers alike, "Herbal Strategies Against Viruses" is an indispensable resource that enables them to fully utilize the therapeutic potential of botanicals in the fight against viral illnesses.

CHAPTER I

Overview of viral infections and their global impact

Role of herbal medicine in viral defense

The hunt for efficient methods to prevent viral infections has long been a priority in medical practice and research. Herbal medicine has been a significant player in this field in recent years, providing various plant-based treatments that may have antiviral qualities. Herbal therapy, in contrast to traditional medications, utilizes the natural substances available in plants to treat illnesses. This comprehensive approach to viral defense includes enhancing the body's innate immune responses in addition to managing symptoms. This section aims to examine the various aspects of herbal medicine's function in viral defense, including its historical foundation, scientific basis, clinical uses, and potential future developments.

Since humans learned that plants could cure a variety of ailments, including viral infections, human societies have long relied on the medicinal properties of plants. To cure infectious diseases, indigenous tribes all over the world have created complex herbal medicine systems by utilizing the knowledge that has been passed down through the years. Many herbal remedies with antiviral qualities are used in traditional medical systems like Traditional Chinese Medicine (TCM), Ayurveda, and Native American medicine. These ancient systems provide a comprehensive framework for viral defense by emphasizing the idea of reestablishing harmony and balance within the body to support resilience against infections and promote health.

Scientific studies conducted in the modern era have confirmed the effectiveness of herbal remedies in treating viral infections and have illuminated the mechanisms behind these remedies' antiviral effects. Numerous plants have bioactive substances with a range of pharmacological characteristics, such as anti-inflammatory, immunomodulatory, and antiviral activities. In experimental settings, it has been demonstrated that certain plants, such as echinacea, garlic, and ginger, have direct virucidal characteristics that prevent viral reproduction and lower viral load. Furthermore, certain herbs have immunostimulatory properties that increase the synthesis of cytokines and immune cell activity to provide a strong defense against viral invaders.

Herbs' abundant phytochemical content offers a supply of antiviral solid substances that can target different phases of the viral replication cycle. Herbs contain bioactive components such as flavonoids, polyphenols, alkaloids, and terpenoids that work through various methods to demonstrate antiviral action. For example, flavonoids that interfere with viral attachment and fusion processes, such as quercetin and kaempferol, impede viral entry and reproduction. Garlic's main ingredient, allicin, inhibits the formation of viral proteins and blocks viral enzymes to produce antiviral effects. Furthermore, a complex blend of bioactive ingredients is frequently found in herbal formulations, which may work in concert to improve efficacy and lower the likelihood of viral resistance.

Further evidence supporting the use of herbal medicine in viral defense has come from clinical research and epidemiological data, which show the herb's potential to both prevent viral infections and lessen the intensity and duration of viral symptoms. For example, extract from elderberries (Sambucus nigra) has been found in randomized controlled trials to shorten the duration of influenza symptoms and lessen the need for conventional treatments. Likewise, it has been demonstrated that Andrographis paniculata, also referred to as the "king of bitters," reduces respiratory viral infection symptoms and speeds up healing. Furthermore, astragalus (Astragalus membranaceus) and licorice root (Glycyrrhiza glabra) are two herbal treatments traditionally used to strengthen the immune system and treat viral respiratory tract infections.

There are still obstacles and restrictions preventing herbal medicine from being fully included in conventional medical procedures, even in light of the mounting data demonstrating its effectiveness in virus protection. The inconsistent quality and standardization of herbal products, which can affect their efficacy and safety, is one of the main problems. Concerns over product uniformity and possible contamination arise from the herbal supplement industry's need for regulated control and established production procedures. Furthermore, using herbal medicines with caution and seeking professional counsel is essential because they may worsen underlying health concerns or interfere with conventional pharmaceuticals.

To sum up, herbal medicine plays an important and developing role in the field of viral defense by providing an alternative to traditional antiviral treatments. Herbal remedies for viral infections are still being investigated and proven to have therapeutic value, from traditional Chinese medicine to contemporary scientific studies. By utilizing the wide range of bioactive substances present in plants and their incorporation into all-encompassing healthcare approaches, we can leverage the natural remedies found in nature to enhance our resistance to viral infections and foster overall health. In the years to come, herbal medicine is expected to become more and more crucial in the fight against infectious diseases as research advances and our understanding grows.

Importance of herbal strategies in combating viral infections

Many civilizations worldwide have long used herbal remedies to prevent and cure various illnesses, including viral infections. In view of the global issues that viral infections pose, the benefits of employing herbal medicines to treat them have recently become apparent. From their accessibility and cost to their potential efficacy and low side effects, these natural therapies have a lot to offer.

The accessibility of herbal remedies for viral infections is one of their main benefits. A significant section of the populace has easy access to and a local source for many of these herbs. In contrast to pharmaceutical treatments, which could necessitate prescriptions or access to medical facilities, herbal remedies are frequently obtained from nearby markets, gardens, or even nature. This accessibility makes sure that people have a practical way to get treatment and preventative measures, especially in environments with limited resources.

In addition, herbal remedies are frequently less expensive than traditional pharmaceutical ones. Herbal treatments are a cost-effective choice for individuals and communities, especially in areas with limited healthcare resources or financial constraints, because their production and delivery costs are often lower. This affordability factor is critical to guaranteeing that everyone in society has access to primary healthcare interventions regardless of financial situation.

In addition to being easily obtainable and reasonably priced, herbal remedies have the potential to be effective in treating viral infections. Several plants have been shown in scientific investigations to have antiviral effects; some of these herbs have shown promising outcomes against a range of viral infections. For instance, studies have been conducted on the potential of herbs like Echinacea, elderberry, ginger, and garlic to boost immunity and prevent viral reproduction. These organic substances have antiviral solid properties because they target many phases of the viral life cycle, such as attachment, entrance, replication, and release.

Furthermore, herbal therapies frequently have a good safety profile with few side effects when used as directed. In contrast to synthetic pharmaceuticals that have the potential to cause various adverse reactions and drug interactions, herbal remedies are typically regarded as safer and more palatable for humans. This is particularly beneficial for vulnerable populations, such as young children, older people, and expecting moms, when lowering the likelihood of unfavorable outcomes is imperative.

Herbal remedies have direct antiviral effects in addition to being essential for promoting general health and immune system performance. Numerous herbs have immunomodulatory properties, which means they can improve the body's capacity to fight viral infections by regulating and bolstering the immune response. Moreover, a number of herbs are high in vitamins, antioxidants, and other bioactive substances that support general health and well-being. People can strengthen their immune systems and lessen their vulnerability to viral infections by including these herbs in their everyday regimen.

But it's important to understand that herbal remedies are not a cure-all and that the quality of the herbal preparation, the particular virus, and individual traits can all affect how effective a herbal strategy is. Furthermore, although herbal medicines can be used in conjunction with conventional medical therapies, they should never be used in place of evidence-based medical interventions, especially in cases that are serious or life-threatening. The safe and successful integration of herbal techniques into conventional healthcare procedures requires cooperation between practitioners of traditional herbal medicine and contemporary healthcare providers.

In summary, it is impossible to overestimate the value of herbal remedies in the fight against viral infections. These natural cures provide accessible, reasonably priced, and possibly beneficial solutions for people and communities worldwide, offering a comprehensive approach to health and well-being. Through the utilization of nature's pharmacy, we can fortify our resistance against viral infections and advance the well-being and adaptability of both individuals and communities.

CHAPTER II

Understanding Viruses

Basics of virology. structure, classification, and replication

Virology, a discipline nestled within the realm of microbiology, is tasked with unraveling the mysteries surrounding viruses and their structure, classification, and replication mechanisms. At its foundation, understanding the structure of viruses is paramount. These microscopic entities typically harbor a core of genetic material, either DNA or RNA, encased within a protective protein shell called a capsid. In certain instances, viruses may also possess an outer lipid envelope acquired from the host cell. The diversity in virus structure is immense, reflecting their ability to infect various hosts and tissues.

Classification of viruses is a complex endeavor, often considering their genetic makeup, morphology, mode of transmission, and host specificity. This taxonomy leads to grouping viruses into families, genera, and species, providing a framework for studying their biology and evolution. The Baltimore classification system, introduced by Nobel laureate David Baltimore, further organizes viruses into seven distinct groups based on their nucleic acid type and replication strategy. It offers insights into the intricate mechanisms viruses propagate within host cells.

Replication, the quintessential hallmark of viruses, underscores their parasitic nature and reliance on host machinery for survival and proliferation. The viral replication process is meticulously orchestrated, beginning with attaching viral surface proteins to specific receptors on host cells. This initial interaction, which can happen through endocytosis or direct fusion with the cell membrane, facilitates viral entry into the cell. Once inside, the virus must navigate the intricate landscape of the host cell to unleash its genetic payload. For DNA viruses, replication often entails the transcription of viral genes into mRNA, followed by translation into viral proteins, and ultimately, viral DNA replication. In contrast, RNA viruses must transcribe their RNA genomes into mRNA using viral polymerases before proceeding to protein synthesis and genome replication. These replication strategies vary widely among different virus families and are a testament to the remarkable adaptability of viruses in exploiting host resources for their benefit.

Beyond mere replication, viruses have evolved intricate mechanisms to evade host immune responses and ensure their survival. Certain viruses conceal themselves in membranes derived from the host to avoid detection, while others encode proteins that disrupt immunological signaling pathways within the host. Additionally, the high mutation rates exhibited by many RNA viruses enable rapid adaptation to changing environments and immune pressures, fostering the emergence of new viral variants with enhanced virulence or transmissibility.

Understanding these evasion strategies is critical for developing effective antiviral therapies and vaccines capable of thwarting viral infections.

Moreover, virology is a cornerstone in the fight against emerging infectious diseases and global pandemics. The ongoing threat posed by viruses such as influenza, HIV, Ebola, and most recently, SARS-CoV-2 underscores the importance of continuous research and surveillance in virology. Advances in molecular virology, structural biology, and immunology have paved the way for developing novel antiviral drugs and vaccines, offering hope in the battle against viral pathogens. Furthermore, interdisciplinary collaborations between virologists, epidemiologists, clinicians, and public health officials are essential for devising strategies to mitigate the spread of viral diseases and safeguard global health security.

In conclusion, the basics of virology encompass a broad spectrum of knowledge ranging from virus structure and classification to replication mechanisms and viral pathogenesis. Through interdisciplinary efforts and technological advancements, scientists continue to unravel the complexities of viral biology, paving the way for innovative approaches to combat viral diseases. To protect public health and lessen the effects of viral outbreaks globally, a thorough grasp of virology is still essential as we traverse the obstacles presented by newly developing infectious pathogens.

Transmission routes and infection mechanisms

Understanding infectious illnesses' pathophysiology and transmission pathways is essential for developing preventative and control measures in public health. Transmission routes and infection processes are critical components of this understanding. Pathogens can spread through a variety of channels, each having unique traits and consequences for managing disease. When diseases are transferred from an infected person to a vulnerable host by physical contact, such as skin-to-skin contact or sexual activity, this is known as direct contact transmission. The spread of illnesses, including HIV/AIDS, STIs, and skin infections, is significantly aided by this mechanism of transmission.

Conversely, germs can spread through contaminated surfaces or items through indirect contact transmission. Consuming food or water tainted with infectious organisms is another typical example, as does touching contaminated surfaces and subsequently contacting your face. Maintaining good sanitation and hand hygiene is essential to preventing illnesses from spreading through indirect contact.

Airborne transmission is the spread of infectious organisms through the atmosphere, which enables people to breathe them in and may result in respiratory diseases. This transmission form is essential for spreading COVID-19, TB, and influenza. Like airborne transmission, droplet transmission is caused by bigger respiratory droplets released when an infected person talks, sneezes, or coughs. These droplets have the ability to spread quickly and directly among people in close quarters, aiding in the spread of illnesses, including bacterial meningitis, the common cold, and some forms of pneumonia. When infections are spread from infected vectors—such as mosquitoes, ticks, or fleas—to humans by blood-feeding, this is known as vector-borne transmission. Diseases like dengue fever, malaria, Lyme disease, and Zika virus infection are spread by this mode of transmission, underscoring the need for vector control strategies in the prevention of disease.

It is crucial to investigate the mechanisms by which viruses infect hosts and cause disease and comprehend the transmission routes. The initial phase of the multi-step infection process often involves the attachment of pathogens to host cells or mucosal surfaces. Adhesins are molecules on the pathogen's surface that connect with corresponding receptors on host cells to enable adherence. Pathogens may infiltrate host tissues and cells after adhesion, which enables them to multiply and disseminate throughout the body. Toxins and other virulence factors that aid in the breach of host barriers and tissue colonization are frequently secreted during invasions. Once within the host, viruses might use a variety of strategies to thwart or avoid the immune system. These include immunological suppression, in which pathogens obstruct immune cell or cytokine activity to reduce immune responses, and antigenic variation, in which pathogens modify their surface proteins to avoid identification by the immune system.

Moreover, several pathogens have developed defense mechanisms to avoid being entirely recognized by the host's immune system. For instance, intracellular pathogens can conceal themselves inside host cells, protecting themselves from immune monitoring. Examples of these pathogens are Mycobacterium tuberculosis and certain viruses. Others, such as HIV, target, and damage essential immune system elements, like CD4+ T cells, impairing the host's capacity to mount a successful defense. Pathogens and the host's immune system interact in a dynamic way, with both parties continuously developing new tactics to obtain the upper hand in the conflict between infection and immunity.

Finally, it should be noted that knowledge of infectious disease transmission pathways and infection mechanisms is crucial to public health initiatives aimed at halting and preventing the spread of infectious illnesses. By identifying the various pathways of transmission and elucidating the mechanisms by which pathogens infect hosts and evade immune detection, researchers and public health officials can develop targeted interventions to halt the spread of transmissible illnesses and lessen their impact on the world's population. Furthermore, research into emerging pathogens and developing novel treatments and vaccines are essential to address present and future infectious disease issues. By having a thorough grasp of the pathways by which infections spread and how they are caused, we can better prepare ourselves to fight infectious diseases and safeguard public health both today and in the future.

Impact of viral infections on public health

Globally, viral infections impact individuals, communities, and entire populations, posing severe challenges to public health systems. These diseases, which can be brought on by a number of viruses, including the flu, HIV, Ebola, Zika, and most recently, COVID-19, can have a significant impact on socioeconomic stability, healthcare infrastructure, morbidity, and mortality. The potential for viral diseases to spread quickly throughout communities and cause pandemics and epidemics is one of the main causes of concern. Viral transmission can occur through a variety of routes, including respiratory droplets, direct contact with bodily fluids, infected surfaces, and vectors like mosquitoes or ticks. Given how easily viruses can spread, it is crucial to implement strong public health policies to stop and manage the spread of viral illnesses.

The strain that viral infections exert on healthcare systems is one of the most direct effects they have on public health. Viral disease outbreaks frequently overwhelm medical institutions, resulting in a scarcity of staff, medical supplies, and hospital beds. The burden on resources may impede the standard of care given to patients, worsening the outbreak's severity and raising death rates. Furthermore, the surge in virally infected individuals may cause delays in the usual course of medical care, including the identification and treatment of other illnesses.

Furthermore, viral infections may have a lasting negative impact on a person's health and well-being. Numerous viruses can result in long-lasting illnesses that last for years or even a lifetime. Prolonged viral infections can compromise the immune system, induce progressive organ damage, and increase the risk of certain cancers. Examples of these infections include the human papillomavirus (HPV), the human immunodeficiency virus (HIV), and hepatitis B and C. These long-term health consequences not only place a heavy burden on those who are affected, but they also raise issues for society in terms of disability and lost productivity, as well as healthcare expenses.

Viral infections can affect one's health directly as well as have significant social and financial repercussions. Infectious illness outbreaks may cause travel restrictions, school closings, quarantine requirements, and disruption of corporate activities. Even while these steps are required to stop the virus from spreading, they may negatively impact trade, employment, education, and overall economic stability. These disturbances frequently disproportionately affect vulnerable populations, such as marginalized groups and low-income communities, aggravating already-existing disparities.

Moreover, stigma, discrimination, and social unrest might result from the uncertainty and dread surrounding viral outbreaks. Individuals afflicted with or linked to a particular virus may experience social exclusion from their communities, impeding attempts to manage the infection's transmission and obtain crucial medical care. In addition to hindering public health initiatives to support preventative measures like immunization and safe sexual practices, stigmatization can also prolong the cycle of transmission.

A multimodal strategy that includes community involvement, diagnosis, treatment, prevention, and surveillance is necessary to respond to viral infections effectively. One of the most effective strategies for stopping viral infections and lessening their effects on the general public's health is vaccination. High levels of population immunity gained by vaccination programs can effectively contain outbreaks and even eliminate certain viruses, as the successful eradication of smallpox and the near-eradication of polio and measles in many regions of the world attest to.

Public health initiatives must prioritize early epidemic detection and control via reliable surveillance systems, quick response mechanisms, and immunization. Preventing the spread of viruses within communities requires the prompt identification of cases, contact tracing, isolation of sick individuals, and application of infection control measures. Furthermore, funding the creation of novel antiviral medications, diagnostic tools, and vaccines is essential to enhancing our capacity to prevent and cure viral infections successfully.

Public health policies that aim to control viral infections must also include education and communication as essential elements. Giving people accurate information about the virus's characteristics, its spread, ways to avoid it, and the available healthcare services can enable them to make decisions about their health and take the necessary precautions to keep others and themselves safe. Collaboration and community engagement with local stakeholders, such as civil society organizations, healthcare professionals, and community leaders, are critical to establishing collective resilience against viral outbreaks, mobilizing resources, and establishing trust.

To sum up, viral infections pose a serious risk to public health and have a wide range of effects on people, groups, and societies. The current COVID-19 epidemic is a sobering reminder of the value of readiness, watchfulness, and cooperation in combating the risks associated with infectious diseases. We can lessen the effects of viral infections and create a healthier, more resilient world for coming generations by putting a priority on prevention, surveillance, and response initiatives, funding research and innovation, and advocating for fairness and social justice.

CHAPTER III

The Science of Herbal Medicine

Historical perspective on herbal remedies for viral infections

Throughout human history, herbal treatments have been widely used in cultures all over the world to cure a wide range of illnesses, including viral infections. A rich tapestry of inherited cultural customs, empirical observations, and traditional knowledge is revealed when considering herbal treatments from a historical viewpoint. The use of plants and herbs as medicinal agents against viral infections has continued from ancient civilizations to modern ones, frequently entwined with spirituality, folklore, and empirical wisdom.

In their writings and manuscripts, ancient civilizations, including the Egyptians, Greeks, Chinese, and Indians, described the usage of medicinal plants to treat a variety of ailments, including viral infections. Herbal medicines are mentioned in the Ebers Papyrus, an ancient Egyptian medical text that dates back to 1550 BCE, for a variety of illnesses, including those brought on by viral viruses. Similar to this, Hippocrates, the Greek physician, promoted the use of antiviral herbs such as elderberry, thyme, and garlic. Traditional Chinese herbal medicine, which included components like ginger, licorice, and astragalus, was utilized to treat viral illnesses like the common cold and influenza in the past. Because of their antiviral qualities, Indian traditional medicine, or Ayurveda, also promotes the use of herbs, including tulsi, neem, and turmeric.

Herbalism was very popular in Europe during the Middle Ages. Herbalists and monks kept gardens full of therapeutic plants, many of which were used to cure common viral illnesses like smallpox and influenza. Herbal medicines were based on traditional knowledge passed down through the generations and empirical observations. They were commonly delivered as tinctures, poultices, or teas. However, traditional herbal medicines rapidly lost popularity in Western nations with the development of modern medicine and the growth of pharmaceuticals in the 19th and 20th centuries.

Nonetheless, herbal treatments continue to be the mainstay of treatment for viral infections in many parts of the world, particularly in areas with little access to contemporary healthcare. In places like China, India, and many African nations, traditional healers still play a crucial role in the delivery of healthcare services. They frequently use herbal medications in their procedures. Furthermore, a fresh understanding of the effectiveness of herbal treatments in treating viral infections has resulted from the current rise of interest in natural and alternative therapies.

Many medicinal plants and herbs have been shown to have antiviral effects by scientific studies undertaken in the last few decades. Herpes simplex virus, respiratory syncytial virus, influenza, and other viruses have been demonstrated to be susceptible to the antiviral activity of compounds present in plants, including ginger, garlic, echinacea, and elderberry. These natural substances are attractive possibilities for the creation of antiviral treatments because they frequently target different phases of the viral replication cycle, such as viral attachment, entrance, replication, and release.

Furthermore, the holistic approach of herbal medicine—which recognizes the interconnection of the body, mind, and spirit—finds resonance with a large number of individuals seeking alternatives to traditional therapy. Herbal treatments frequently seek to bolster the immune system, assist the body's natural healing processes, and help the patient regain harmony and balance. Furthermore, some plants and herbs have symbolic worth beyond their therapeutic qualities due to their cultural relevance and spiritual connotations, which enhances the healing process even more.

Ultimately, the historical analysis of herbal treatments for viral infections emphasizes the long-standing significance of plants and herbs in medical procedures. The application of herbal medicine has been influenced by scientific research, empirical findings, and cultural traditions from ancient civilizations to the present. Traditional herbal medicines continue to provide insightful information and therapeutic alternatives for treating viral disorders, even in spite of the significant progress modern medicine has made in treating viral infections. Integrating the wisdom of ancient herbal medicine with current scientific knowledge may pave the way for more holistic approaches to healthcare and wellness as we traverse the challenges of infectious diseases in the twenty-first century.

Pharmacological principles of botanical medicine

Phytotherapy, or herbal medicine, is another name for botanical medicine, which has been used for ages in many different civilizations. It entails using plants and products derived from plants to cure, prevent, or lessen a range of medical ailments. The various chemical compounds present in plants, each with distinct biological activities and therapeutic potentials, constitute the foundation of the pharmacological concepts underpinning botanical medicine. These guidelines cover the recognition, extraction, preparation, and delivery of plant-based medicines to utilize their pharmacological properties efficiently.

The identification of plant-active ingredients that confer therapeutic benefits is a cornerstone of botanical medicine. Alkaloids, flavonoids, terpenoids, and phenolic compounds are only a few of the many chemical compounds found in plants. These bioactive ingredients have pharmacological effects that support their therapeutic actions by interacting with the body's physiological systems. Alkaloids from the opium poppy (Papaver somniferum), for instance, have analgesic solid effects because they attach to opioid receptors in the central nervous system and alter how painful something feels.

Moreover, according to botanical medicine, standardization and quality control are crucial for guaranteeing the uniformity and effectiveness of herbal medicines. Quantifying the quantity of particular active ingredients in herbal remedies is known as standardization, and it aids in batch-to-batch uniformity and dose calculation. To maintain the integrity and potency of plant materials, quality control measures include botanical identification, growth practices, harvesting techniques, processing processes, and storage conditions.

Botanical medicines frequently show synergistic effects in addition to individual elements, which might be attributable to the intricate interactions among various molecules within the plant matrix. This phenomenon, called the "entourage effect," implies that, in comparison to isolated substances, the combined action of many elements may improve treatment effects. For example, the synergistic interplay of cannabis (Cannabis sativa) terpenes, flavonoids, and cannabinoids results in a variety of pharmacological effects, such as analgesia, anti-inflammatory action, and mood and appetite modification.

Furthermore, knowledge of botanical medications' therapeutic benefits and possible side effects depends heavily on their pharmacokinetic and pharmacodynamic features. Pharmacokinetics is the study of how herbal components enter the body and how their distribution, metabolism, excretion, and absorption affect their bioavailability and duration of action. The term "pharmacodynamics" describes plant components' physiological and biochemical impacts on specific target tissues or organ systems, clarifying their modes of action and potential therapeutic applications.

The mode of administration greatly influences the pharmacokinetic profile of botanical medications. Oral intake is the most popular way, although depending on the intended therapeutic result and the properties of the plant constituents, other techniques like topical application, inhalation, and intravenous infusion are also used. For instance, the volatile oils found in peppermint (Mentha piperita) are frequently breathed to reduce nausea and enhance mental clarity, while extracts of arnica (Arnica montana) are applied topically to provide anti-inflammatory and analgesic benefits.

Furthermore, while using botanical medications in clinical settings, it is crucial to consider their safety and possible side effects. Natural does not always mean safe, although a lot of botanicals have a long history of traditional use and safety profiles that are known. Adverse responses, however, can happen, especially in cases of incorrect dosing, herb-drug combinations, or individual vulnerability. Therefore, pharmacovigilance is essential for keeping an eye on and documenting unfavorable occurrences related to the use of botanical medicines in order to protect patient safety and enhance therapeutic results.

To sum up, the pharmacological principles of botanical medicine include a thorough grasp of substances produced from plants, standardization, and quality control, synergistic interactions, pharmacokinetics and pharmacodynamics, route of administration, and safety considerations. By incorporating these concepts into clinical practice, medical professionals can effectively utilize the therapeutic potential of botanical medicines while maintaining patient safety and high standards of care. Botanical medicine is developing as an essential part of integrative healthcare with continued study and evidence-based treatment, providing a range of therapeutic choices for the promotion of health and well-being.

Evidence-based approach to herbal antiviral activity

The investigation of herbal remedies to treat viral infections has attracted a lot of attention in recent years. A growing number of people are interested in the possible antiviral qualities of different herbs due to the advent of novel viral threats and the shortcomings of traditional antiviral medicines. The centuries-old practice of using plants for medicinal purposes is the foundation of this quest for herbal antiviral activity, which is combined with contemporary scientific techniques meant to confirm their effectiveness. In order to determine the safety and effectiveness of herbal medicines against viral infections and clarify the mechanisms of action, in vitro studies, animal trials, and clinical research are all part of the evidence-based approach to herbal antiviral activity.

Investigating the bioactive substances found in medicinal plants is a crucial component of the evidence-based approach to herbal antiviral efficacy. Numerous herbs include compounds such as flavonoids, alkaloids, terpenoids, and polysaccharides that are known to have antiviral effects. These substances show a variety of modes of action, such as boosting cellular defense systems, modifying immunological responses, and preventing viral replication. Researchers can isolate, characterize, and assess the antiviral activity of these bioactive compounds against a variety of viruses, including coronaviruses, herpes simplex virus, influenza, and human immunodeficiency virus (HIV), using in vitro experiments.

Furthermore, evaluating the effectiveness of herbal treatments in vivo requires careful consideration of animal trials. The pharmacokinetics, biodistribution, and toxicity characteristics of isolated chemicals or herbal extracts can be better understood by using animal models. Researchers can monitor the impact of herbal medicines on survival rates, viral load, and illness progression in animals infected with certain viruses. These preclinical investigations aid in the prioritization of candidates for additional clinical research and advance our knowledge of the therapeutic potential of herbal therapies.

The evidence-based approach's cornerstone is clinical research, which offers vital information on the efficacy and safety of herbal antiviral treatments when applied to human patients. RCTs, or randomized controlled trials, are used to assess how well herbal medicines work therapeutically in comparison to mainstream antiviral therapies or placebo. These trials evaluate variables like the degree of symptoms, length of sickness, side effects, and virus clearance. Additionally, by combining the available data and spotting patterns in numerous studies, observational studies and systematic reviews/meta-analyses provide insightful information.

Challenges still need to be addressed in the field of herbal antiviral therapy despite encouraging results from preclinical and clinical studies. The challenges of standardizing herbal products are still significant because different plant species, growing environments, harvesting strategies, and preparation procedures exist. Maintaining uniformity in the composition and potency of herbal extracts is crucial for their efficacy and reproducibility. Furthermore, in clinical practice, issues about possible side effects, long-term safety, and herb-drug combinations should be carefully considered.

The evidence-based approach to the antiviral properties of herbal remedies highlights the significance of fusing traditional wisdom with modern scientific techniques. Researchers can find novel antiviral drugs and maximize their therapeutic application by fusing scientific examination with the knowledge of traditional herbal medicine. In order to fully understand herbal remedies and their potential to treat viral infections, collaboration between virologists, pharmacologists, botanists, and physicians is essential.

The evidence-based strategy for herbal antiviral activity is a harmonious combination of conventional knowledge and cutting-edge scientific research. By means of methodical inquiry that encompasses in vitro testing, animal investigations, and clinical trials, scientists endeavor to clarify the antiviral mechanisms of herbal treatments and assess their therapeutic effectiveness. Although there are still issues with safety, standardization, and clinical integration, the development of herbal antiviral medication has excellent potential to expand our defenses against viral infections. Adopting this multidisciplinary strategy will promote innovation and broaden the range of antiviral treatments that may be made using the extensive collection of medicinal plants.

CHAPTER IV

Key Botanicals with Antiviral Properties

Overview of potent antiviral herbs

Throughout history, people have used natural treatments found in nature to treat a wide range of illnesses, including viral infections. Utilizing medicinal plants' antiviral properties for therapeutic purposes has garnered renewed attention in recent years. These herbs have bioactive solid components, making them a promising therapeutic and preventative option for viral infections. Many antiviral herbs are available, but a few stand out for their exceptional efficacy and safety records.

Purple coneflower, or Echinacea purpurea, is well known for strengthening the immune system. Echinacea, abundant in flavonoids, polysaccharides, and alkamides, has antiviral solid properties by inducing the development of immune cells like T-cells and macrophages. Research has demonstrated that echinacea extracts can prevent the spread of many viruses, such as the herpes simplex virus and the influenza virus.

Licorice root (Glycyrrhiza glabra) is prized in traditional medicine systems for its many therapeutic properties, which include antiviral solid properties. Polysaccharides and saponins found in astragalus have direct antiviral properties and support the immune system. Studies reveal that astragalus extracts can prevent the growth of many viruses, such as respiratory syncytial virus, hepatitis, and influenza.

Glycyrrhiza glabra, or licorice root, is highly prized in traditional medical systems for its many therapeutic properties, which include solid antiviral actions. Glycyrrhizin, the active ingredient, exhibits inhibitory actions against various viruses, such as respiratory viruses, herpes simplex virus, and HIV. Additionally, licorice root has immune-modulating properties that increase its effectiveness as an antiviral medication.

In addition to being valued for its fragrant flavor in cooking, oregano (Origanum vulgare) possesses antiviral solid qualities. Two substances with well-known antibacterial and antiviral properties found in oregano essential oil include carvacrol and thymol. Research has demonstrated that oregano oil can prevent the growth of multiple viruses, such as the norovirus and respiratory syncytial virus.

For centuries, people have appreciated garlic's culinary and therapeutic benefits (Allium sativum). Allicin, the primary bioactive ingredient in garlic, possesses potent antiviral qualities against a range of viruses, including influenza, rhinovirus, and respiratory syncytial virus. Garlic also strengthens the immune system, which makes it an effective weapon against viral diseases.

Zingiber officinale, or ginger, is another herb that has been shown to have antiviral qualities. The bioactive components of ginger, namely gingerol and school, have strong antiviral properties against respiratory viruses like respiratory syncytial virus and influenza. Additionally, ginger has anti-inflammatory properties that help reduce the symptoms of viral infections.

Renowned for its relaxing qualities, lemon balm (Melissa officinalis) also possesses antiviral solid capabilities. By interfering with viral enzymes, the active ingredient rosmarinic acid prevents the spread of viruses. The effectiveness of lemon balm extracts against the herpes simplex virus and other enveloped viruses has been demonstrated.

To summarize, research into potent antiviral herbs provides a viable treatment option for viral illnesses. Nature's defense against viruses includes echinacea, astragalus, licorice root, oregano, garlic, ginger, and lemon balm, to name just a few. These herbs offer complete protection against viral infections by enhancing immunity and preventing viral multiplication. Including these herbs in regular diet and wellness regimens could provide a safe, all-natural way to boost antiviral defenses and advance general health and well-being.

Mechanisms of action and bioactive compounds

The investigation of natural substances and their methods of action has become a crucial field of study in modern science. Numerous plants, animals, and microorganisms contain bioactive chemicals, which have a wide range of impacts on biological systems, from harmful to medicinal. Comprehending the complex mechanisms by which these molecules function is essential to maximizing their potential for a range of uses in food science, agriculture, and medicine.

Bioactive substances comprise a wide range of molecules, such as phenolics, alkaloids, flavonoids, and terpenoids. These substances engage in a variety of mechanisms of interaction with biological systems, frequently focusing on certain cellular functions or molecular pathways. For example, opioid receptors in the central nervous system are the site of binding for alkaloids like morphine, which modify pain perception. Comparably, flavonoids—which are found in large amounts in fruits and vegetables— showcase antioxidant qualities by eliminating oxidative stress and scavenging free radicals, which lessens cellular damage linked to a number of ailments.

Bioactive chemicals function through methods that go beyond fundamental receptor interactions, including intricate molecular pathways and cellular signaling cascades. Numerous bioactive substances act as activators or enzyme inhibitors, controlling vital metabolic processes necessary for maintaining cellular homeostasis. For instance, the polyphenols in green tea reduce cholesterol levels and have the cardioprotective effect of inhibiting the action of enzymes involved in lipid metabolism.

Furthermore, some bioactive substances change the structure of chromatin and have an impact on transcriptional activity in order to modify gene expression through epigenetic mechanisms. The preventive and curative measures of disease are greatly impacted by the ability to regulate gene expression, particularly in the case of cancer, where aberrant gene expression is necessary for the development and spread of tumors.

Furthermore, when ingested simultaneously, bioactive substances show antagonistic or synergistic interactions that can intensify or decrease biological effects. The "food matrix effect," as this phenomenon is called, emphasizes how crucial it is to consider dietary patterns and food combinations when evaluating the potential health effects of bioactive substances. For example, consuming antioxidant-rich fruits and vegetables coupled with dietary fat sources increases the bioavailability of fat-soluble antioxidants, enhancing their potential health benefits.

Apart from their possible medical applications, bioactive substances are essential for farming and food storage. Phytoalexins, for example, are plant-derived substances that act as organic insecticides, shielding plants against microbes and other pests. Similar to this, aromatic essential oils derived from plants possess antibacterial properties that hinder the development of foodborne infections and extend the shelf life of perishable food items. In addition to lowering dependency on artificial pesticides and antibiotics, the use of bioactive compounds in agriculture encourages environmentally and financially sound sustainable farming methods.

Even though bioactive chemicals have great promise for medical and agricultural applications, it is essential to consider any potential negative consequences. If ingested in excess, certain substances may have cytotoxic or genotoxic effects that could be harmful to human health. Furthermore, interactions between drugs and bioactive substances may have unforeseen effects that change the effectiveness and metabolism of the drugs. Thus, thorough safety evaluations and legislative actions are necessary to guarantee the responsible use of bioactive chemicals in a variety of applications.

To sum up, the investigation of mechanisms of action and bioactive substances is an exciting area of scientific inquiry with significant ramifications for food science, agriculture, and human health. Researchers can harness the therapeutic potential of natural substances while minimizing potential hazards by deciphering the intricate connections between bioactive molecules and biological systems. In the end, the creation of innovative treatments, sustainable farming methods, and better food options will be made more accessible by the integration of cutting-edge technologies and multidisciplinary approaches, all to the benefit of society at large.

Traditional and modern uses of selected botanicals

Since ancient times, botanicals have been used for various reasons in human society, from medicinal to gastronomic and cultural. The use of botanicals has changed, including contemporary scientific discoveries and conventional wisdom. This section highlights the significance of certain botanicals in various facets of human life by examining their historical and contemporary use.

Ginger (Zingiber officinale), used for ages in ancient medical systems like Ayurveda and ancient Chinese Medicine (TCM), is one of the most well-known herbs. Ginger is valued in traditional medicine for its digestive qualities and is frequently applied to relieve motion sickness, nausea, and indigestion. It's also thought to have antioxidant and anti-inflammatory qualities. Many of these traditional benefits have been supported by research in the modern era. For example, studies have shown how effective ginger is at reducing inflammation and easing nausea. Ginger has also entered contemporary cooking, giving food taste and depth. Its extract is also used in several pharmaceutical and cosmetic items.

Curcuma longa, or turmeric, is another plant with a long history of traditional use. It is a common ingredient in Indian food and Ayurvedic treatment. Research has shown that curcumin, an amino acid found in turmeric, exhibits both anti-inflammatory and antioxidant properties. Traditional medicine has used turmeric to treat a number of illnesses, including gastrointestinal problems, rheumatoid arthritis, and skin ailments. Many of these traditional uses have been validated by modern research, with multiple studies showing curcumin's ability to enhance overall health and manage inflammatory illnesses. Due to its alleged health benefits, people are adding turmeric tablets to their daily routines, which has increased its popularity in the contemporary wellness industry.

The olive tree (Olea europaea), cultivated for millennia, holds a special place in Mediterranean culture. Extra virgin olive oil, sourced from the fruit of the olive tree, occupies a significant role in Mediterranean cuisine, primarily due to its numerous health-promoting properties. In traditional medicine, olive oil has been employed both topically for addressing skin and hair issues and orally for its potential cardiovascular advantages. Recent research has revealed a multitude of health advantages linked to the consumption of olive oil, including a decreased likelihood of heart disease, inflammation, and specific cancer types. Furthermore, olive leaf extract, made from the olive tree's leaves, has drawn interest due to its possible antioxidant and immune-boosting qualities, making it appealing to contemporary customers looking for natural solutions for wellbeing.

Cannabis (Cannabis sativa) is one plant that has become very popular in both traditional and modern settings. For thousands of years, cannabis has been utilized for both medical and recreational purposes, as evidenced by historical records from ancient civilizations such as the Chinese and Egyptians. Cannabis was used in traditional medicine to heal a variety of illnesses, lessen inflammation, and ease pain. Cannabinoids, like THC and CBD, have been found to have a variety of effects on the body as a result of extensive research into the medicinal potential of cannabis in modern times. Many areas now have legal access to medical cannabis for the treatment of multiple sclerosis, epilepsy, chronic pain, and other ailments. Furthermore, the non-psychoactive cannabis ingredient CBD has gained enormous popularity due to its supposed ability to soothe and reduce anxiety. As a result, many items in the wellness market include CBD.

In conclusion, traditional knowledge has formed the basis for modern scientific investigation for millennia, and botanicals have been essential to human health and civilization. The four chosen plants covered in this section—cannabis, ginger, turmeric, and olive oil— showcase the range of conventional and contemporary use and their ongoing significance in various spheres of human endeavor. Botanicals will undoubtedly continue to play a significant role in our knowledge of and application of medicine and lifestyle as long as society adopts holistic approaches to health and wellness.

CHAPTER V

Herbal Strategies for Common Viral Infections

Influenza and respiratory viruses

Every year, influenza and respiratory viruses cause a great deal of morbidity and mortality, which is a significant public health concern worldwide. Influenza viruses, mainly kinds A and B of the Orthomyxoviridae family, cause influenza, also called the flu. These viruses are infamous for their quick mutations, which can cause seasonal outbreaks and sporadic pandemics with extensive effects. The respiratory system is the main target of influenza viruses, which can cause symptoms ranging from mild respiratory distress to severe pneumonia and, in rare circumstances, even death.

Apart from influenza, other respiratory viruses that cause respiratory illnesses are adenovirus, human metapneumovirus (hMPV), respiratory syncytial virus (RSV), and coronaviruses like the Middle East respiratory syndrome coronavirus (MERS-CoV), and the severe acute respiratory syndrome coronavirus (SARS-CoV)., along with the common cold, contribute to respiratory illnesses. Although these viruses' pathophysiology and genomic structure vary, they are primarily transmitted through respiratory droplets formed during talking, sneezing, and coughing.

With laboratory testing, reliable identification of influenza and other respiratory viral diseases can be more accessible due to their typical clinical appearance. Fever, coughing, sore throats, nasal congestion, body aches, and exhaustion are typical symptoms. Certain viruses, however, may have unique characteristics. For example, RSV infections typically cause more severe symptoms in newborns and early childhood. On the other hand, coronaviruses, like SARS-CoV-2, can result in a variety of symptoms, including gastrointestinal issues, neurological issues, and loss of taste and smell.

Proactive measures, prompt diagnosis, and suitable treatment plans are essential for managing respiratory viral diseases, including influenza. The mainstay of influenza protection continues to be vaccination, with yearly vaccine programs aimed at certain virus strains expected to be prevalent in the forthcoming flu season. Furthermore, non-pharmaceutical measures, including mask-wearing, social distancing, respiratory etiquette, and hand cleanliness, are successful in lowering the spread of viruses, especially during pandemics and outbreaks.

Antiviral drugs are essential for treating influenza, particularly in patients at high risk or very sick. When used early in an infection, medications such as oseltamivir and zanamivir can help minimize symptoms, shorten the length of sickness, and lower the risk of consequences. Nonetheless, the rise in antiviral resistance highlights the necessity of continued monitoring and the creation of innovative therapeutic approaches.

Novel respiratory viruses like SARS-CoV-2 have emerged recently, posing unheard-of difficulties for international health systems. The COVID-19 pandemic, brought on by SARS-CoV-2, highlighted how linked today's globe is and how crucial it is to have effective planning and response plans. The development of novel treatment modalities, such as monoclonal antibodies and antiviral medications, as well as the quick deployment of vaccinations, have resulted from the exceptional acceleration of efforts to create COVID-19 vaccines, therapies, and diagnostics.

Influenza and respiratory viruses still constitute a serious threat to public health despite advancements in prevention and treatment, especially for vulnerable groups like the elderly, small children, pregnant women, and people with underlying medical disorders. To improve public health policies and methods to limit the burden of respiratory viral infections, ongoing research efforts are crucial to understanding viral pathogenesis, host immune responses, and viral evolution.

In conclusion, respiratory viruses and influenza represent a vast family of pathogens that can dramatically raise morbidity and death rates worldwide. A multifaceted strategy is necessary for effective prevention and management techniques, including vaccination, non-pharmaceutical interventions, prompt diagnosis, and proper use of antiviral drugs. Moreover, tackling new risks and enhancing readiness for pandemics and outbreaks in the future depends on continued research and international cooperation.

Herpes simplex virus (HSV)

Millions of people worldwide are impacted by the ubiquitous infectious agent known as herpes simplex virus (HSV). It falls into one of two categories. HSV-2 and HSV-1. HSV-2 usually causes genital herpes, but HSV-1 is mainly linked to oral herpes, which can result in fever blisters or cold sores. Different mucosal surfaces can be infected by either kind of HSV, which can result in a variety of clinical symptoms. The majority of HSV infections remain lifelong, and they occasionally reactivate to cause symptomatic outbreaks.

Direct contact with infected lesions or bodily fluids is how HSV is spread. While HSV-2 is mainly spread through sexual contact, HSV-1 is typically spread through oral-to-oral contact. Nonetheless, oral-genital contact might allow either type to spread to either area. Furthermore, during birthing, vertical transfer from mother to neonate can happen, which could cause severe issues for the newborn.

HSV becomes latent in the sensory nerve ganglia after the first infection and can remain there for the duration of the host. The virus may occasionally reactivate, causing recurring symptom outbreaks. Conditions like stress, disease, hormone fluctuations, and UV radiation can bring on reactivation. Reactivation is the process by which the virus returns to the original infection site by traveling via nerve fibers, causing symptoms to reappear.

The symptoms of an HSV infection can vary significantly in their clinical manifestations, from painful lesions to asymptomatic shedding. Primary infections frequently cause more severe symptoms, such as fever, enlarged lymph nodes, and excruciating ulcers. While recurring outbreaks are typically milder and last less time, they can be upsetting and uncomfortable. Moreover, immune system-compromised patients may encounter more frequent and severe breakouts.

Diagnostic procedures for HSV infection usually include laboratory tests and clinical assessment. Although the diagnosis is frequently made based on the patient's history and clinical presentation, laboratory testing such as serological assays, polymerase chain reaction (PCR), and viral culture can confirm the diagnosis. Additionally, serological testing can identify the HSV type (1 or 2) and evaluate a person's immunological state.

Antiviral medication and supportive care are part of managing HSV infection. Antiviral drugs like valacyclovir, famciclovir, and acyclovir are frequently administered to suppress viral shedding and transmission, in addition to lessening the intensity and duration of symptoms. Important aspects of care also include supportive measures like pain management, good cleanliness, and counseling regarding the risk of transmission.

A variety of tactics, such as antiviral prophylaxis, safer sexual practices, and education, are necessary to prevent the spread of HSV. Those who are known to be infected with HSV should inform their sexual partners of their status and use barrier techniques like condoms to lower the chance of transmission. Antiviral drugs can also be used as suppressive therapy to lower the likelihood of transmission in people who experience outbreaks frequently or in couples who are discordant.

Despite advancements in diagnosis and treatment, herpes simplex virus (HSV) continues to pose a significant public health challenge due to its widespread occurrence and detrimental effects on individuals' quality of life. Ongoing research aims to create innovative treatment approaches, such as vaccinations, to stop primary infections and lessen the impact of recurring epidemics. Additionally, in order to de-stigmatize HSV and encourage safer sexual practices in the community, ongoing education and awareness initiatives are crucial.

In summary, millions of people worldwide are afflicted with the widespread viral infection known as herpes simplex virus (HSV). It is linked to a variety of clinical presentations, ranging from painful lesions to asymptomatic shedding. Clinical assessment and laboratory tests are used for diagnosis, while antiviral medication and supportive care are used for treatment. Antiviral prophylaxis, safer sexual practices, and education are examples of prevention tactics. Notwithstanding obstacles, there is promise for better future HSV infection prevention and treatment, thanks to ongoing research and public health initiatives.

Human immunodeficiency virus (HIV)

With millions of victims worldwide, the Human Immunodeficiency Virus (HIV) remains one of the most dangerous international health problems. HIV is a type of retrovirus known as a lentivirus. It attacks the immune system, primarily CD4 cells, which are essential for the body's defense against infections. The primary modes of virus transmission include biological fluids such as blood, semen, vaginal secretions, and breast milk. HIV does not spread through familiar touches, such as handshakes or hugs, but it can be transmitted through sexual contact, sharing of needles, and mother-to-child during childbirth or breastfeeding.

HIV multiplies quickly once it enters the body, weakening the immune system. The most severe form of HIV infection, acquired immunodeficiency syndrome (AIDS), is brought on by this immune system deterioration. People who have AIDS are more vulnerable to malignancies and opportunistic infections that a healthy immune system would typically be able to fight off. HIV infection develops into AIDS without proper treatment, significantly raising the chance of death.

The fact that HIV can go years without showing any symptoms and hence remain undetected is one of the virus's most worrisome characteristics. Many people might not become aware that they are infected until they start to exhibit symptoms, which can take years to appear. Frequent early signs of HIV infection include rash, lymph node swelling, fever, and exhaustion. These symptoms, though, are not exclusive to HIV and are frequently confused with those of other diseases.

Antiretroviral therapy (ART) has significantly altered the way that HIV infection is treated. In order to successfully suppress viral replication and allow the immune system to heal, antiretroviral therapy (ART) combines several drugs that target distinct stages of the HIV lifecycle. When administered appropriately and consistently, antiretroviral therapy (ART) can considerably lower the body's viral load, halting the spread of HIV to AIDS and greatly extending the lives of those infected with the virus. ART is an essential part of HIV prevention initiatives since it can also lower the risk of HIV transmission to uninfected partners.

Even with the tremendous advancements in HIV prevention and treatment, a number of obstacles still exist. There is still a disparity in access to HIV testing, care, and treatment, especially in low- and middle-income nations where resources may be few. Testing and treatment adherence are still hampered by stigma and prejudice against people living with HIV, which keeps many people from getting the care they require. In addition, new problems, including medication resistance and the survival of HIV reservoirs in the body, provide continuous difficulties for HIV research and treatment development.

The prevention of HIV infection is essential to halting its spread. Pre-exposure prophylaxis, or PrEP, has shown to be a very successful preventive measure when used in conjunction with other interventions, such as encouraging safe sexual practices, condom access, and harm reduction techniques for drug injectors. Pre-exposure prophylaxis, or PrEP, involves taking an antiviral pill on a regular basis to lower the risk of HIV infection in those who are at high risk of getting the virus. Moreover, lowering transmission rates and enabling people to take charge of their sexual health depends on initiatives to de-stigmatize HIV, encourage testing, and offer thorough sexual education.

To sum up, HIV continues to be a serious worldwide health concern with wide-ranging effects on society, the economy, and public health. The HIV epidemic still disproportionately affects underprivileged communities and underserved populations despite advances in prevention and treatment. To indeed halt the HIV epidemic, it is imperative to address the many factors that contribute to the virus's spread and to guarantee that everyone has fair access to care, treatment, and testing. We may work toward a time when HIV does not endanger the health and welfare of people everywhere by conducting ongoing research, integrating communities, and adopting preventative actions.

Hepatitis viruses

Hepatitis viruses impact millions of individuals globally, presenting a severe threat to global health. Hepatitis is typified by inflammation of the liver, which can result in cirrhosis of the liver and cancer, among other health issues. Hepatitis A, B, C, D, and also E are among the various groups into which hepatitis viruses can be divided. The symptoms, means of prevention, and modes of transmission of each kind vary.

The primary way that the hepatitis A virus (HAV) spreads is through contaminated food or drink. Additionally, intimate contact with an infected individual or sexual interaction might spread it. Acute sickness caused by a HAV infection usually manifests as exhaustion, nausea, abdominal discomfort, and jaundice. But the majority of Hepatitis A cases go away on their own without resulting in permanent liver damage. The best defense against contracting Hepatitis A is vaccination, particularly for visitors to regions where the virus is highly prevalent.

Contact with contaminated blood, semen, or other body fluids can spread the hepatitis B virus (HBV). Sexual contact, sharing syringes or needles, or mother-to-child transmission during childbirth can all result in this. Acute and chronic HBV infections are possible; persistent infections raise the risk of malignancy and liver cirrhosis. Hepatitis B can cause joint pain, weariness, jaundice, and stomach discomfort. Since vaccinations are so successful in halting the spread of Hepatitis B, they should be administered to all neonates and high-risk individuals.

Hepatitis C virus (HCV) is primarily transmitted through sharing needles or getting blood transfusions from infected donors among individuals who come into contact with blood. Chronic HCV infection frequently results in liver damage over time. Many Hepatitis C patients may go years or even decades without showing any symptoms. When symptoms do appear, they could be as follows: joint pain, jaundice, weariness, and stomach discomfort. Hepatitis C cannot be prevented. However, antiviral drugs can successfully treat the virus and lower the risk of liver damage.

The hepatitis D virus (HDV) is a flawed virus that needs HBV to proliferate. HDV infection can develop as a superinfection in those who already have HBV infection or concurrently with HBV infection. Like HBV, HDV is spread through contact with contaminated blood or other body fluids. When combined with HBV infection, HDV infection can cause liver damage that is more severe. Preventing HBV infection through immunization and other preventive methods is essential to preventing HDV infection.

The primary way that the hepatitis E virus (HEV) spreads is through contaminated food or water, especially in developing nations with subpar sanitary infrastructure. HEV infection usually results in acute sickness with symptoms resembling those of other viral hepatitis types. The majority of Hepatitis E cases go away on their own without resulting in permanent liver damage. Although there isn't a vaccine for hepatitis E at the moment, transmission can be avoided by practicing better sanitation and hygiene.

In summary, hepatitis viruses are a broad class of pathogens with a range of symptoms, means of transmission, and defense mechanisms. Hepatitis A and

B infections can be avoided with vaccination, while chronic Hepatitis C management requires antiviral drugs. To stop the spread of Hepatitis E, hygiene and sanitation standards must be improved, especially in places with inadequate infrastructure for sanitation. In order to battle the global burden of viral hepatitis and lessen its impact on public health, increased awareness, early detection, and prompt intervention are essential.

Emerging viral threats and pandemics

Global health security is constantly challenged by emerging viral threats and pandemics, which pose severe risks to human populations and economies around the globe. Although infectious diseases have plagued humans throughout history, the modern world's fast globalization and interconnection have accelerated the emergence and dissemination of novel viruses. The current COVID-19 epidemic is a sobering reminder of how susceptible our international health system is to dangers of this nature. In order to lessen their effects and stop future pandemics, it is essential to comprehend the characteristics of newly emerging viral risks, their sources, the dynamics of transmission, and the appropriate response tactics.

Emerging viral hazards are characterized by their unpredictable nature. Because viruses may change and adapt, there are always new risks to the public's Health. Viruses known as zoonotic—those that infect people after starting in animals—are hazardous. Spillover events—in which viruses spread from animals to humans—are more likely to occur when natural ecosystems are invaded, when wildlife is traded, and when intensive farming methods are used. Such zoonotic transmissions are the source of several recent pandemics, such as COVID-19, SARS, and HIV/AIDS. For this reason, early identification and intervention depend heavily on tracking and comprehending the dynamics of animal reservoirs and human-animal interfaces.

Emerging viral hazards can travel across borders more quickly as a result of globalization and increased travel. Because of the interconnection of the world, a pandemic that starts in one area can spread rapidly to other parts of the world. Mass gatherings, trade, and air travel all offer ways for infectious agents to spread quickly. A virus can spread over international borders in a matter of weeks, as the COVID-19 pandemic illustrates, underscoring the necessity of concerted international efforts for pandemic preparedness and response. It takes coordinated public health measures, prompt information sharing, and early identification to contain outbreaks and stop them from spreading into pandemics.

Emerging viral hazards have an impact on economics, cultures, and geopolitical environments in addition to public Health. Supply chains are disrupted, healthcare systems are strained, and social inequality is made worse by pandemics. Millions of people have been forced into poverty, and trillions of dollars have been lost in GDP as a result of the COVID-19 epidemic alone. Pandemics disproportionately affect vulnerable groups, such as the elderly, the immunocompromised, and marginalized communities. Furthermore, pandemics can exacerbate pre-existing tensions and erode public confidence in institutions by igniting social unrest and political instability. Therefore, reducing the complex effects of pandemics requires fostering resilience at the individual, community, and governmental levels.

A multidisciplinary approach that incorporates medical, scientific, social, and political components is necessary for an effective response to developing viral threats. For readiness, funding research and development of medications, vaccines, and diagnostics is essential. Enhancing the public health infrastructure—which includes lab networks, surveillance systems, and hospital capacity—is equally crucial. Moreover, encouraging global solidarity and cooperation is crucial for taking collective action against pandemics. Global preparedness and response capacities are improved by initiatives like the World Health Organization's (WHO) Global Outbreak Alert and Response Network (GOARN), which enables the quick deployment of resources and knowledge during outbreaks.

Addressing the root causes of viral emergence, such as deforestation, urbanization, and climate change, is essential to averting future pandemics. Reducing the likelihood of zoonotic spillover events requires the implementation of sustainable land use practices, biodiversity conservation, and responsible wildlife management. Furthermore, encouraging One Health strategies that acknowledge the interdependence of environmental, animal, and human Health is crucial for reducing the threat of new viral infections. Strategies centered around One Health can help anticipate and prevent future pandemics before they worsen by promoting collaboration across sectors and specialties.

To sum up, pandemics and new viral threats present intricate problems that call for thorough and well-coordinated solutions. Although viruses are unpredictable and can cause significant difficulties, preventive steps can lessen their effects and stop future outbreaks from becoming worldwide emergencies. Humanity can improve its resistance to newly emerging infectious diseases and protect the Health and welfare of future generations by funding research, fortifying healthcare systems, encouraging international cooperation, and tackling the underlying causes of viral emergence.

CHAPTER VI

Herbal Formulations and Preparation Methods

Herbal teas, tinctures, and extracts for viral defense

Herbal medicines have become a tempting way to strengthen the body's defenses against viruses, especially in light of viral epidemics and the continued search for effective preventive measures. Plant-based medicines, including herbal teas, tinctures, and extracts, represent a wide variety of botanical therapies that have been utilized for ages in several cultures all over the world. In viral defense, these natural formulations offer a wide range of bioactive substances recognized for their antiviral qualities, offering an alternative to traditional medicine.

Herbal teas are a calming and healing way to strengthen the immune system. They are made from dried leaves, petals, seeds, or roots of medicinal plants. Due to their abundance of flavonoids, antioxidants, and other phytochemicals, plants like ginger, echinacea, and elderberry are well known for strengthening the immune system. For example, echinacea has shown promise in improving immune function by promoting the maturation of white blood cells, which are necessary in battling against infections caused by viruses. Similarly, strong anthocyanins found in elderberry tea have antiviral properties that hinder viral reproduction and alter immune responses when applied to influenza viruses.

Convenient and effective herbal therapy is provided via tinctures and concentrated herbal extracts produced by macerating plant material in glycerin or alcohol. Herbal extracts, including those from licorice root, astragalus, and olive leaves, are highly valued for their antiviral characteristics and capacity to bolster the body's defense mechanisms.

By preventing viral replication and having immunomodulatory properties, licorice root extract, which contains glycyrrhizin and glycyrrhetinic acid, exhibits antiviral efficacy against a variety of viruses, including respiratory syncytial virus and herpes simplex virus. Astragalus tincture, made from the roots of the Astragalus membranaceus plant, helps the body fight against viral invaders by boosting the activity of natural killer cells and macrophages, which in turn boosts the immune system. Furthermore, by inhibiting viral attachment to host cells and replication, olive leaf extract, which is high in polyphenols like oleuropein, works against a variety of viruses, including respiratory viruses like influenza and rhinovirus.

Concentrated solutions from plant ingredients extracted with a solvent, known as herbal extracts, provide a powerful defense against viral infections. Herb extracts, like those from Andrographis paniculata, garlic, and oregano, have antiviral solid qualities because of their varied phytochemical makeup. Allicin and other sulfur-containing chemicals found in garlic extract have broad-spectrum antiviral effects by preventing viruses' growth and their entry into host cells. Rich in phenolic compounds including thymol and carvacrol, oregano extract exhibits strong antiviral properties against respiratory viruses like respiratory syncytial virus and rhinovirus. Its mechanism involves the suppression of viral replication and modulation of immune responses. Additionally, Andrographis extract, derived from the leaves and stems of Andrographis paniculata, contains andrographolide, a bioactive compound with robust antiviral and immunomodulatory properties. It's been demonstrated that andrographis extract prevents the growth of several viruses, such as the dengue and influenza viruses, and boosts immunity by promoting phagocytosis and producing more interferons.

In summary, many natural therapies for bolstering the body's resistance against viral infections may be found in herbal teas, tinctures, and extracts. These botanical treatments are essential allies in the ongoing fight against infectious diseases because they are abundant in bioactive chemicals that have antiviral qualities. Using the therapeutic potential of medicinal plants, we can strengthen our defenses against viral threats and improve immunological function safely and efficiently. Including herbal medicine in our toolkit of knowledge about managing viral outbreaks is a promising way to support people's resilience and overall health when faced with hardship.

Synergistic herbal blends and formulations

Herbal medicine techniques employ a holistic approach to health and wellness, which is embodied in synergistic herbal blends and formulations that combine traditional knowledge with contemporary technology. These are carefully prepared concoctions of different herbs that have been carefully chosen and combined to complement one another's healing qualities and offer a wide range of health advantages. Synergistic herbal formulations, which are based on the idea that a whole is stronger than the sum of its parts, use the synergistic interactions of several herbs to produce effective treatments for a variety of medical conditions.

The idea that each plant has a distinct biochemical makeup and medicinal qualities is fundamental to synergistic herbal mixes. In order to develop blends that treat many aspects of health and enhance overall well-being, herbalists, and formulators carefully pick herbs with complementary actions and qualities. Herbs with immuno-stimulating, anti-inflammatory, and antioxidant qualities, for instance, can be combined in a combination intended to improve immune function, strengthen the body's natural defenses, and encourage resilience against infections and illnesses.

The idea of synergy—the combination of two or more components that produce an impact more extensive than the sum of their individual effects—is one of the fundamental ideas guiding the design of synergistic herbal blends. Synergy can take many different forms in herbal therapy, such as increased therapeutic efficacy, better absorption, and decreased side effects. Herbalists can maximize each ingredient's therapeutic potential and create more comprehensive and effective formulations by combining plants with synergistic activities.

Taking energetics—the innate properties and traits of herbs that affect their effects on the body—into account is another essential part of making synergistic herbal mixes. Herbs are classified by energy qualities, such as hot, cold, moist, or dry, in ancient herbal medicine systems like Ayurveda and ancient Chinese Medicine (TCM). Herbalists seek to promote optimal health and vitality by harmonizing the body's internal environment and balancing these energies within a blend. For instance, a combination meant to support digestive health might contain cooling herbs to balance excess heat and alleviate inflammation and warming herbs to encourage digestion.

Another important consideration in the creation of synergistic herbal blends is dosage and quantity. Herbalists have to carefully balance the proportions of each herb to get the intended medicinal effect without adding too much or lessening the blend's effectiveness. Certain herbs possess greater potency or more potent effects than others, requiring proportional changes to guarantee well-balanced and efficient compositions. The dosage and absorption of herbal blends can also be affected by the way they are administered, such as teas, tinctures, capsules, or topical applications. This emphasizes the significance of carefully formulating and dosing herbal mixes.

While creating synergistic herbal blends, safety must always come first because some herbs might worsen preexisting medical issues, mix negatively with drugs, or react negatively in those who are already sensitive. When preparing blends for therapeutic use, herbalists must carefully evaluate each herb's safety profile and any potential contraindications and safety requirements. Furthermore, maintaining the effectiveness of herbal formulations and protecting consumer health depend on the quality and purity of the substances used in herbal products.

In conclusion, by combining the complimentary properties of numerous herbs, synergistic herbal formulations and blends provide a thorough approach to health and wellness. This results in effective and comprehensive therapies. Herbalists and formulators can carefully choose and combine herbs with complementary actions and qualities to create blends that treat various aspects of health and enhance general well-being. Synergistic herbal blends, which provide safe, efficient, and comprehensive answers for today's health issues, are based on the concepts of synergy, energetics, dose, and safety. They are a prime example of how traditional wisdom and scientific innovation are integrated in the field of herbal medicine.

Dosage guidelines and safety considerations

In order to guarantee the efficacy and security of medicine administration, dosage recommendations and safety factors are essential. Achieving therapeutic results while lowering the chance of side effects requires careful dosage administration. Based on predetermined parameters, healthcare professionals—including doctors, nurses, and pharmacists—determine the proper dosage for each patient.

Usually, these recommendations are predicated on the patient's age, weight, health, and hepatic or renal function. To maximize patient safety, factors including medication interactions, contraindications, and possible adverse effects must also be taken into mind.

A cornerstone of dose administration is the idea of "start low, go slow." This method places a strong emphasis on starting therapy at a low dose and titrating it up gradually in accordance with the patient's reaction. Healthcare professionals can determine the patient's tolerance and modify the dosage to meet therapeutic objectives while lowering the possibility of adverse effects by starting cautiously. When administering medications with restricted therapeutic windows or a high potential for toxicity, vigilance is essential.

Additionally, unique suggestions for patient demographics, including pediatric, geriatric, pregnant, or nursing patients, are frequently included in dose guidelines. Specific populations might have certain physiological traits or vulnerabilities that call for specific dose modifications. For instance, weight-based dosing may be necessary for juvenile patients in order to accommodate for variations in body mass and metabolism, and age-related changes in renal or hepatic function may result in decreased drug clearance in elderly patients. Medication safety must also be carefully considered by expectant and nursing mothers in order to reduce prenatal exposure and potential harm to the nursing child.

Healthcare practitioners have to be alert about possible drug interactions in addition to taking patient-specific considerations into account. Numerous drugs may interact with one another in ways that change how effective they are or raise the possibility of adverse side effects. Many processes, such as pharmacokinetic interactions (e.g., modification of drug metabolism or excretion) and pharmacodynamic interactions (e.g., additive or synergistic effects), can lead to drug-drug interactions. To reduce risks and improve treatment outcomes, healthcare providers need to be aware of possible interactions and consult trustworthy sources such as medication interaction databases or pharmacists.

Safety concerns include more than just dosage estimates and drug interactions; they also include using the proper methods to administer medications. To avoid mistakes and guarantee patient safety, healthcare providers must follow defined procedures for the production, storage, and administration of medications. This includes confirming prescription orders, double-checking computations, appropriately labeling drugs, and using the proper administration methods. Additionally, patient education is necessary to encourage drug compliance and provide patients the confidence to manage their own health actively.

Medication errors can still happen even with strict adherence to safety procedures and dose requirements because of a variety of issues, such as human error, malfunctioning systems, and poor communication. As a result, healthcare institutions need to put pharmaceutical solid safety measures in place, like prescription reconciliation procedures, barcode medication administration, and computerized physician order entry (CPOE). These tactics seek to lower the frequency of mistakes, increase medicine delivery accuracy, and eventually improve patient outcomes.

To sum up, safety concerns and dosage recommendations are essential parts of medicine administration procedures. Healthcare professionals can maximize therapeutic outcomes while limiting the risk of side effects by following established dosage recommendations. To further ensure patient safety, it is crucial to carefully evaluate patient-specific characteristics, medication interactions, and appropriate medication administration strategies. By employing a multidisciplinary strategy that incorporates clinical knowledge, technology developments, and patient education, medical practitioners can reduce risks and encourage the safe and efficient use of medications.

CHAPTER VII

Integrative Approaches to Viral Defense

Complementary use of herbal medicine with conventional treatments

The amalgamation of herbal medicine and conventional treatments has been the subject of growing attention and acknowledgment in global healthcare practices. The complementary use of herbal treatments presents a promising path for addressing a variety of health conditions and improving therapeutic outcomes, even while conventional medication continues to be the cornerstone of modern healthcare. This method, which is also known as integrative medicine, combines the best aspects of herbal and conventional therapy to give patients all-encompassing, individualized care. Herbal medicine is a rich heritage that spans ages and many civilizations. It is drawn from plants and natural sources. Its reputed safety, accessibility, and all-encompassing tenets make it appealing. Conventional medicine, on the other hand, places a strong emphasis on the use of technology, standardized procedures, and rigorous scientific validation to identify and cure diseases. Healthcare professionals can take advantage of the synergistic potential to maximize patient well-being and treatment efficacy by combining various approaches.

The ability to reduce side effects and improve therapeutic results is one of the main benefits of combining herbal medicine with conventional therapies. The potential for adverse effects, pharmacological combinations, and tolerance problems with conventional drugs generally limits their long-term usefulness. In contrast, herbal therapies are prized for their ability to support general health and energy and for acting in a comparatively mild manner. Herbal therapy has the potential to reduce side effects, increase treatment tolerance, and facilitate the body's inherent healing mechanisms when used prudently in conjunction with conventional medicines. For example, when treating ailments like arthritis, herbal supplements like ginger and turmeric may be used in addition to prescription anti-inflammatory pharmaceuticals to provide further symptom alleviation and lessen the need for high-dose prescriptions.

Herbal medicine's holistic approach also fits with the expanding understanding of how mind, body, and spirit are intertwined in health and wellness. Herbal treatments frequently address not just the symptoms but also the underlying causes of sickness by promoting systemic harmony and resolving underlying imbalances. Patients looking for more individualized, patient-centered care find resonance with this holistic approach, which encourages empowerment and participation in their recovery process. Herbal therapy integration with traditional medicine promotes a more holistic approach to healthcare, where natural remedies, lifestyle changes, and prevention are valued in addition to medicinal interventions.

Herbal medicine used in conjunction with conventional medicines can improve treatment outcomes, increase therapeutic alternatives, and close gaps in the healthcare system. Conventional herbal medicines can treat illnesses for which conventional medications may be ineffective or unavailable. They provide a wide range of medicinal substances with different modes of action. Certain botanicals, such as Valerian root and St. John's Wort, have shown promise in the treatment of mild to moderate depression and anxiety. This offers patients who might not get the desired effect from conventional antidepressants or who would instead use natural therapies as an alternative. Healthcare providers have access to a more excellent range of resources when these herbal therapies are incorporated into treatment programs, which enables more customized and flexible patient care procedures.

Moreover, the amalgamation of traditional medical practices with herbal medicine emphasizes the significance of evidence-based practice and cooperation among medical practitioners. Despite having a long empirical history, herbal medicine still needs constant investigation and rigorous scientific confirmation before it can be effectively incorporated into modern healthcare practices. To assess the safety, effectiveness, and best practices for using herbal medicines in addition to conventional treatments, cooperation between researchers, herbalists, and conventional practitioners is vital. Integrative medicine fosters a more inclusive and all-encompassing approach to healthcare delivery by bridging the gap between conventional wisdom and modern research, which is advantageous to both patients and practitioners.

The supplementary use of herbal medicine in conjunction with conventional treatments has potential benefits, but there are drawbacks that need to be taken into account as well. Standardized quality control, dose recommendations, and consumer and healthcare provider education are crucial among them. Herbal medications, unlike pharmaceutical drugs, differ greatly in terms of their potency, purity, and composition, which raises questions regarding consistency and safety. To guarantee the dependability and safety of herbal remedies and reduce the possibility of contamination, adulteration, or mislabeling, regulatory control, and quality assurance procedures are crucial. In order to handle the intricacies of herbal medicine, including possible herb-drug interactions, contraindications, and patient counseling, healthcare personnel must also complete training and education.

In summary, the integration of herbal medicine and conventional treatments is a promising paradigm in contemporary healthcare that maximizes patient care by combining their respective capabilities. Through the utilization of herbal treatments in conjunction with conventional medications, healthcare providers can improve treatment outcomes, increase therapeutic alternatives, and advance a more comprehensive approach to patient care. However, in order to fully utilize integrative medicine, coordinated efforts are needed to meet quality assurance, regulatory compliance, and educational requirements. Integrative medicine has the potential to transform the way healthcare is delivered and give patients the tools they need to reach their best possible health and wellness with more research, cooperation, and dedication to evidence-based practice.

Holistic strategies for immune support and viral prevention

Global awareness of the significance of avoiding viral infections and preserving a robust immune system has increased recently. While excellent vaccinations and treatments for a variety of viruses have been made possible by medical science developments, it is still critical to employ holistic approaches for immune support and viral prevention. Comprehensive lifestyles that support mental, emotional, and spiritual health in addition to physical health are embraced by holistic approaches. Through the integration of many activities and behaviors, individuals can enhance their immune system and reduce their vulnerability to viral infections.

Nutrition is essential for both preventing viruses and boosting the immune system. A diet full of complete, nutrient-dense foods supplies vital vitamins, minerals, and antioxidants for the best possible immune system performance.

To ensure adequate intake of immune-stimulating nutrients like zinc, vitamins D and C, and omega-3 fatty acids, it is important to include a diverse range of foods in the diet. This includes fruits, vegetables, whole grains, lean meats, and healthy fats. Limiting processed meals, sugar-filled drinks, and heavy alcohol use also aids in lowering inflammation and boosting immune system function.

Another crucial element of comprehensive immune support and viral prevention is regular physical activity. Exercise boosts immune system performance, strengthens the body, and improves cardiovascular health. Exercises that are moderate in intensity, like swimming, cycling, or brisk walking, increase the production of immune cells and antibodies and lessen the vulnerability to viral infections. Regular exercise to maintain a healthy weight also increases immunity in general and lowers the risk of chronic illnesses linked to immune dysfunction.

Getting enough sleep is essential for immune system maintenance and viral protection. The body goes through vital processes of regeneration and repair as you sleep, such as the synthesis of antibodies and cytokines that fight illnesses. Lack of sleep over an extended period of time impairs immune function and makes people more vulnerable to viral infections. Viral resistance and immunological function can be strengthened by prioritizing quality sleep and implementing a regular bedtime routine, a sleep-friendly atmosphere, and screen time limits before bed.

An essential part of comprehensive immune support is the use of stress management strategies. Extended periods of stress impair immunity and compromise the body's capacity to fend against diseases. Integrating techniques that help lower stress levels, such as yoga, tai chi, deep breathing exercises, or mindfulness meditation, can lessen the adverse effects of stress on the immune system. Developing resilience and embracing positivity also strengthen the immune system and improve the body's capacity to handle viral threats.

Maintaining good hygiene practices is crucial in preventing the spread of viral diseases. Hands should always be washed with soap and water to properly rid them of bacteria and viruses, especially prior to consuming food or touching the face. It's advised to use hand sanitizers with at least 60% alcohol content when handwashing facilities aren't available. Furthermore, two other ways to practice respiratory hygiene are limiting the spread of respiratory viruses like coronaviruses and influenza by concealing coughs and sneezes with tissues or your elbow and avoiding direct contact with sick people.

Including immune-stimulating herbs and vitamins can support all-encompassing approaches to virus avoidance. Many plants, such as echinacea, elderberry, garlic, and ginger, have immune-boosting and antiviral qualities. These herbal medicines can be added to teas, tinctures, or supplements to boost immune function and lessen the intensity and duration of viral infections. Medical professionals must be consulted before taking new supplements to guarantee safety and effectiveness.

Finally, building social ties and a feeling of community supports immunological resilience and general well-being. Robust social support systems boost immunity, ease emotional distress, and lower stress levels. Developing connections, participating in community events, and deepening relationships all contribute to mental and emotional well-being, fortifying the body's resistance against viral infections.

In summary, comprehensive approaches to immune support and virus prevention take a multimodal approach that takes into account several facets of health and wellness. People can increase their immunity and reduce the risk of viral infections by maintaining good hygiene, taking immune-boosting herbs and supplements, eating a balanced diet, getting regular exercise, getting enough sleep, managing stress, and cultivating social networks. Adopting a holistic lifestyle boosts immunity and encourages general health and vigor, enabling people to flourish in the face of viral obstacles.

Collaborative efforts between herbalists and healthcare providers

Herbalists and medical professionals working together is a new trend that has great promise for improving patient care and fostering holistic well-being. The complementary nature of herbal medicine and conventional healthcare practices has come to light in recent years, and as a result, practitioners from these two fields have begun working together more frequently. The foundation of this partnership is a shared commitment to patient-centered care, honest communication, and respect for one another. Collaborative initiatives seek to improve treatment outcomes, advance health literacy, and provide people the power to make educated decisions about their health by utilizing the unique talents of herbalists and healthcare professionals.

The amalgamation of conventional knowledge and scientifically validated procedures is among the principal advantages of cooperation between herbalists and medical professionals. Herbalists contribute a wealth of information regarding the therapeutic qualities of plants that have been used for years in traditional medicine. Herbalists can share their knowledge of herbal treatments and obtain access to clinical and scientific data that support the safety and effectiveness of different herbal interventions by working with healthcare providers. Combining traditional knowledge with the most modern developments in medicine allows for treatment programs that are tailored to the requirements and preferences of each patient.

Furthermore, joint initiatives between herbalists and medical professionals may close gaps in the provision of healthcare, especially in regions where access to traditional treatments is restricted. Herbal therapy provides complementary therapies for a variety of medical issues, including immunological support, stress-related diseases, and chronic pain and inflammation. Herbalists and medical professionals can increase the therapeutic alternatives accessible to patients by collaborating, ensuring that their varied requirements are satisfied in an inclusive and culturally sensitive way.

Collaboration between herbalists and healthcare professionals not only increases treatment possibilities but also promotes better responsibility and transparency in the practice of herbal therapy. To mitigate the risk of adverse reactions or interactions with conventional pharmaceuticals, healthcare practitioners can collaborate effectively by establishing clear channels of communication and sharing relevant patient information. Professionals with different backgrounds can collaborate to guarantee the safe and efficient application of herbal medicines through multidisciplinary teamwork. By leveraging collective expertise and best practices, they can improve patient outcomes and cultivate a culture of collaboration and continuous learning in healthcare settings.

Moreover, cooperative initiatives between herbalists and medical professionals may advance health literacy and allow patients the confidence to manage their own health actively. Healthcare professionals can assist patients in making well-informed decisions about the inclusion of herbal medicines in their treatment regimens by offering information and resources on herbal medicine. This could entail going over the possible advantages and disadvantages, clearing up common misconceptions, and offering advice on how to use herbal products in a responsible and safe manner. Collaborative efforts seek to promote a sense of autonomy and self-efficacy in patients by equipping them with the knowledge and skills necessary to navigate their healthcare alternatives. In the end, this will result in improved patient satisfaction and health results.

Although there are possible advantages to working together, there are also obstacles that need to be overcome for the partnership between herbalists and medical professionals to be successful. These could include disparities in professional backgrounds and training, different legal systems controlling the use of herbal remedies, and even inconsistencies in therapeutic philosophies or methods. However, by acknowledging and tackling these issues with candid communication, collaborative decision-making, and a dedication to patient-centered care, professionals may get past obstacles and create win-win alliances that improve the standard and accessibility of healthcare for everybody.

To sum up, cooperative efforts between herbalists and medical professionals offer a viable strategy for improving patient care and fostering holistic well-being. Working together, herbalists and healthcare providers can transform the way we deliver healthcare by fusing traditional wisdom with evidence-based practices, increasing treatment options, promoting accountability and transparency, and enabling patients to make educated decisions. By fostering an environment of mutual respect, transparent communication, and a shared dedication to patient-centered care, healthcare professionals can collaborate to enhance treatment outcomes, advance health literacy, and elevate the standard of care for both individuals and communities.

CHAPTER VIII

Herbal Medicine in Pandemic Preparedness

Role of botanicals in pandemic response and preparedness plans

Finding practical methods and techniques to lessen the effects of global health emergencies like pandemics is crucial. While conventional pharmaceuticals play a significant role in combating infectious diseases, there is growing recognition of the potential contributions of botanicals in pandemic response and preparedness plans. Botanicals, derived from plants, have long been utilized for their medicinal properties across various cultures and traditions. Their diverse biochemical compositions offer a rich source of bioactive compounds with therapeutic potential against infectious agents. Incorporating botanicals into pandemic response and preparedness plans can enhance resilience, complement existing strategies, and provide sustainable solutions in combating emerging health threats.

One of the key advantages of botanicals lies in their broad spectrum of bioactive compounds, which possess antiviral, antibacterial, and immunomodulatory properties. Flavonoids, alkaloids, terpenoids, and polyphenols are examples of plant-derived substances that display a variety of biological actions that can reduce the growth of viruses, alter immune responses, and lessen the symptoms of infectious disorders. For instance, botanical extracts containing flavonoids like quercetin and epigallocatechin gallate (EGCG) have demonstrated antiviral activity against respiratory viruses, including influenza and coronaviruses, by interfering with viral entry and replication processes.

Furthermore, botanicals offer a reservoir of natural compounds with potential therapeutic efficacy against drug-resistant pathogens, which pose significant challenges to conventional pharmaceutical interventions. The complex chemical profiles of plants present a diversified approach to combatting microbial resistance, as they often contain multiple bioactive constituents that can target various mechanisms of microbial survival and proliferation. Botanical-based therapies have the ability to overcome resistance mechanisms and provide alternative treatment options for infectious diseases by utilizing the synergistic effects of these chemicals.

Moreover, the utilization of botanicals aligns with principles of traditional and complementary medicine, which emphasize holistic approaches to health and wellness. Many botanical remedies have been traditionally used for their immune-boosting and anti-inflammatory properties, making them valuable assets in strengthening host defenses and reducing the severity of viral infections. Integrating botanical-based interventions into pandemic response plans can facilitate community engagement and acceptance, leveraging cultural knowledge and practices to promote public health resilience.

In addition to their therapeutic potential, botanicals offer advantages in terms of accessibility, affordability, and sustainability, particularly in resource-limited settings. Unlike synthetic drugs, which often require complex manufacturing processes and extensive infrastructure, botanical medicines can be sourced from locally available plants and prepared using simple extraction techniques. This decentralized approach to production and distribution enhances the accessibility of treatments, especially in remote or underserved areas where conventional healthcare services may be limited.

Furthermore, the cultivation and utilization of medicinal plants promote environmental sustainability and biodiversity conservation. Many botanical species used in traditional medicine are cultivated or harvested from wild habitats, emphasizing the importance of ecosystem conservation and sustainable harvesting practices. Pandemic response strategies can serve environmental stewardship and public health objectives by encouraging the cultivation of medicinal plants and bolstering traditional knowledge systems. This fosters resilience and the interdependence of human and ecological health.

However, despite their potential benefits, the integration of botanicals into pandemic response and preparedness plans necessitates rigorous scientific validation, quality assurance, and regulatory oversight. Challenges such as standardization of herbal preparations, assessment of safety and efficacy, and establishment of quality control measures must be addressed to ensure the reliability and reproducibility of botanical-based interventions. Collaborative efforts involving researchers, healthcare professionals, policymakers, and traditional medicine practitioners are essential to navigate these complexities and maximize the contributions of botanicals to pandemic preparedness and response efforts.

In conclusion, botanicals represent valuable assets in pandemic response and preparedness plans, offering diverse bioactive compounds with therapeutic potential against infectious diseases. Their broad spectrum of biological activities, compatibility with traditional medicine systems, accessibility, and sustainability make them promising candidates for complementing conventional pharmaceutical interventions. However, their integration requires comprehensive scientific validation, quality assurance, and regulatory frameworks to ensure safety, efficacy, and reliability. By harnessing the potential of botanicals and fostering interdisciplinary collaborations, we can enhance our resilience to pandemics and build more robust, holistic approaches to global health security.

Community-based initiatives and herbal resources during outbreaks

Herbal remedies and community-based programs are essential for enhancing traditional medical treatments during public health emergencies and outbreaks. These programs efficiently address health issues by utilizing the resources and collective wisdom of communities. For instance, herbal resources have been used for ages for their possible medical benefits in many different civilizations. Communities frequently resort to traditional herbal medicines during outbreaks as affordable and culturally appropriate substitutes. However, effectiveness, safety, and cultural sensitivity must all be carefully considered when incorporating herbal resources into public health programs.

Initiatives rooted in the community make use of available resources and local expertise to contain outbreaks quickly. These programs are based on the ideas of independence and community development. Community-based organizations are essential to the prevention and management of disease because they raise awareness, organize volunteers, and offer assistance to those who are impacted. To guarantee coordinated responses, these efforts frequently work with government organizations and medical specialists. These programs encourage adherence to preventive measures, improve communication, and build trust by actively involving communities.

Throughout history, herbal remedies have played a significant role in conventional medical practices. For thousands of years, people have utilized plants for their medical qualities, and native civilizations frequently have deep knowledge of the regional flora and its uses. Communities may use herbal medicines as readily available and reasonably priced replacements for conventional medicine during outbreaks. Because they are thought to have antibacterial and immune-boosting qualities, plants like ginger, garlic, and turmeric are well- liked options for symptom management and immune system support. Herbal tinctures, poultices, and teas are also frequently used to ease respiratory symptoms, lessen inflammation, and enhance general well-being.

However, there are significant safety, effectiveness, and cultural sensitivity concerns when using herbal resources during outbreaks. While many traditional treatments have undergone extensive testing and are backed by scientific evidence, some have not and could be dangerous if taken incorrectly. Potential issues with using herbal goods include contamination, adverse responses, and herb-drug interactions. In addition, public health communications and treatments need to take cultural variations in health beliefs and behaviors into consideration. To close the gap between conventional wisdom and contemporary science, cooperation between researchers, healthcare professionals, and traditional healers is crucial.

During epidemics, community-based programs are essential for encouraging the long-term usage of herbal remedies. These programs give community people the tools, resources, and education they need to make educated decisions about their health. For example, community herbal gardens are excellent places to grow therapeutic herbs and encourage self-care habits. These programs encourage holistic approaches to health and healing and build community resilience by establishing linkages between people and plants. Furthermore, programs that encourage the sustainable collection, production, and preservation of medicinal plants aid in the preservation of traditional knowledge systems and biodiversity.

To sum up, community-based programs and herbal remedies are essential tools in the battle against epidemics and public health crises. These programs support holistic approaches to health and healing and supplement traditional medical treatments by utilizing the collective knowledge and resources within communities. However, effectiveness, safety, and cultural sensitivity must all be carefully considered when incorporating herbal resources into public health programs. Working together, community organizations, medical professionals, and researchers can optimize the advantages of herbal therapy while reducing its possible drawbacks. Communities can increase health equality, develop resilience, and lessen the impact of outbreaks on vulnerable groups by banding together.

Ethical considerations in the use of herbal medicine during crises

During emergency situations, such as pandemics, natural catastrophes, or other calamities, the use of herbal medicine frequently presents itself as a potentially effective and easily accessible form of therapy. But using herbal therapy in such turbulent times brings up important ethical issues that need to be carefully considered. Although herbal medicine has a long history and is deeply ingrained in culture, it does not have the same level of scientific validation or standardized regulation as conventional medications. Therefore, using herbal treatments in emergency settings raises ethical questions about safety, effectiveness, accessibility, cultural sensitivity, and informed permission.

Safety is one of the main ethical issues when using herbal medicine in emergency situations. In contrast to pharmaceutical pharmaceuticals that undergo rigorous testing and regulatory supervision, the composition, strength, and purity of herbal therapies can differ significantly. Herbal medicines carry a greater danger of adulteration, contamination, and adverse reactions if proper quality control procedures aren't followed. Robust systems for quality assurance are necessary to ensure the safety of herbal therapies during crises. These mechanisms include rigorous sourcing, standardized production processes, and comprehensive toxicity testing.

Furthermore, there is ongoing debate regarding the effectiveness of herbal therapy in meeting particular health demands in times of crisis. Although several herbal medicines have shown therapeutic promise in treating various illnesses, it is still being determined how beneficial they will be in dire circumstances with inadequate infrastructure and resources. Due to ethical constraints, a cautious strategy based on empirical data and clinical research is required for the promotion and implementation of herbal therapies. A thorough scientific examination is necessary to determine if herbal medicines are effective and to stop the spread of unproven claims that could jeopardize public health initiatives in times of emergency.

Another ethical consideration for the use of herbal therapy in times of crisis is accessibility, especially in environments with limited resources. Herbal treatments are frequently accessible, reasonably priced, and culturally appropriate substitutes for traditional medical care. They provide relief to underserved groups that are struggling financially or logistically. Disparities in the availability of herbal knowledge, resources, and traditional treatment methods, however, have the potential to worsen already-existing injustices and disadvantage underprivileged communities. Prioritizing fairness and inclusivity, ethical frameworks governing the use of herbal medicine in crisis response tactics should support programs that enable underprivileged communities to utilize their customary healing methods while removing access obstacles.

A crucial ethical factor to take into account when integrating herbal medicine into crisis management procedures is cultural sensitivity. Deeply ingrained beliefs and traditions are reflected in the extensive knowledge of herbal treatments that many indigenous cultures have inherited throughout the years. Respecting indigenous wisdom and cultural traditions means appreciating the various healing paradigms that are present in various communities. Herbal medicine, in times of crisis, requires a culturally humble, collaborative, and reciprocal ethical response. Indigenous viewpoints must be respected, and traditional healing systems must be included in larger healthcare frameworks with consent and due regard for intellectual property rights.

A critical ethical precept guiding the use of herbal medicine in emergency situations is informed consent, which calls for open communication and patient autonomy. People who are experiencing a crisis may be more susceptible to being taken advantage of, receiving false information, or being forced to utilize herbal medicines, which emphasizes the significance of making educated decisions. It is morally required of healthcare professionals and humanitarian organizations to protect the rights of impacted communities by giving truthful information, encouraging communication, and honoring personal decisions about healthcare options, including the use of herbal medicine in treatment plans.

In conclusion, using herbal medicine in an emergency raises a number of ethical concerns that should all be carefully considered and avoided. Herbal treatments can be easily obtained and culturally appropriate interventions in emergency situations, but maintaining public health demands strict adherence to safety, effectiveness, accessibility, cultural sensitivity, and informed consent standards. Collaborative efforts are necessary to incorporate traditional healing practices into larger healthcare frameworks, address access inequities, and promote equitable, patient-centered care in order to engage with herbal medicine ethically during times of crisis. Stakeholders can prioritize the autonomy and well-being of affected communities while using the curative potential of herbal medicine to support crisis response efforts by adhering to ethical standards and supporting evidence-based approaches.

CHAPTER IX

Herbal Medicine and Immune Support

Enhancing immune function with botanicals

The human immune system is a complex network of cells, tissues, and organs that work together to defend the body against pathogens and maintain overall health. While proper nutrition, adequate sleep, regular exercise, and stress management are essential for optimal immune function, botanicals have gained increasing attention for their potential role in enhancing immune health. Botanicals, derived from plants, have been used for centuries in traditional medicine systems worldwide for their therapeutic properties. These natural compounds contain various bioactive constituents that can modulate immune responses and support the body's defense mechanisms.

One of the most widely studied botanicals for immune enhancement is echinacea. Echinacea, derived from the purple coneflower, contains compounds such as alkamides, polysaccharides, and flavonoids, which have been shown to stimulate immune cells and increase the production of cytokines, proteins involved in regulating immune responses. Research suggests that echinacea supplementation may help reduce the duration and severity of upper respiratory tract infections by bolstering the immune system's ability to fight off invading pathogens.

Another botanical with immune-boosting properties is elderberry. Elderberry, derived from the fruit of the Sambucus nigra plant, is rich in antioxidants, particularly flavonoids such as quercetin and anthocyanins. These compounds possess anti-inflammatory and antiviral effects, which may help reduce the risk of respiratory infections and alleviate symptoms of the common cold and flu. Studies have shown that elderberry supplementation can enhance immune function by increasing the production of cytokines and enhancing the activity of natural killer cells, key players in the body's defense against viral infections.

Turmeric, a bright yellow spice derived from the Curcuma longa plant, is another botanical renowned for its immune-boosting properties. Curcumin, the active compound in turmeric, exhibits potent anti-inflammatory and antioxidant effects, which may help modulate immune responses and promote overall immune health. Research suggests that curcumin supplementation can enhance immune function by stimulating the activity of immune cells, such as T cells and macrophages, and reducing inflammation throughout the body.

Ginseng, a traditional medicinal herb native to East Asia, has also been valued for its immune-enhancing properties. Ginsenosides, the active compounds in ginseng, possess immunomodulatory effects that can strengthen the immune system and improve resistance to infections. Studies have shown that ginseng supplementation may enhance the proliferation and activity of immune cells, enhance antibody production, and increase the body's ability to combat pathogens. Additionally, ginseng has been found to have adaptogenic properties, helping the body cope with stress and maintain homeostasis, which is crucial for optimal immune function.

In addition to these botanicals, several other herbs and plants have been studied for their potential immune-boosting effects, including astragalus, garlic, and medicinal mushrooms such as reishi and shiitake. These botanicals contain bioactive compounds that can modulate immune responses, enhance the body's defense mechanisms, and support overall immune health.

While botanicals offer promising potential for enhancing immune function, it is essential to use them judiciously and under the guidance of a healthcare professional. Some botanicals may interact with medications or have contraindications for certain medical conditions. Furthermore, the quality and purity of botanical supplements can vary significantly, so it is essential to choose reputable brands that adhere to strict quality control standards.

In conclusion, botanicals offer a natural and holistic approach to supporting immune health. With their diverse array of bioactive compounds, botanicals such as echinacea, elderberry, turmeric, and ginseng can help modulate immune responses, reduce inflammation, and enhance the body's ability to fight off infections. Incorporating these botanicals into a healthy lifestyle, along with proper nutrition, adequate sleep, regular exercise, and stress management, can contribute to overall immune resilience and well-being. However, it is crucial to approach botanical supplementation with caution and consult with a healthcare professional to ensure safety and efficacy.

Adaptogenic herbs and stress management in viral infections

The human immune system is a sophisticated network comprising cells, tissues, and organs that play a vital role in preserving overall health and protecting the body against illnesses and infections. Although a healthy diet, enough sleep, regular exercise, and stress reduction are necessary for the best immune system performance, botanicals are becoming increasingly well-known for their possible contribution to immune system enhancement.

Because of their therapeutic qualities, botanicals—derived from plants—have been employed for ages in traditional medical systems worldwide. Numerous bioactive components included in these natural substances have the ability to influence immunological responses and bolster the body's defense systems.

Echinacea is one of the botanicals for immune boosting that has been researched the most. Echinacea, which is a plant related to the purple coneflower, has substances including alkamides, polysaccharides, and flavonoids that have been demonstrated to activate immune cells and boost the synthesis of cytokines, which are proteins that control immunological responses. Research indicates that by enhancing the immune system's capacity to fend off invasive microorganisms, echinacea supplements may help shorten the length and severity of upper respiratory tract infections.

Elderberry is another plant that has immune-boosting qualities. The fruit of the Sambucus nigra plant yields elderberries, which are high in flavonoids such as anthocyanins and quercetin, which are known antioxidants. These substances have antiviral and anti-inflammatory properties that may lessen the chance of respiratory infections and ease the flu and common cold symptoms. According to studies, taking supplements containing elderberries can improve immune function by boosting cytokine synthesis and natural killer cell activity—two essential components of the body's fight against viral infections.

The Curcuma longa plant yields turmeric, a brilliant yellow spice that is also well-known for strengthening the immune system. Turmeric's main ingredient, curcumin, has potent antioxidant and anti-inflammatory properties that may help control immunological responses and improve immune system function as a whole. According to research, taking supplements containing curcumin may improve immune function by lowering systemic inflammation and inducing the activity of immune cells, including macrophages and T cells.

East Asian ginseng, a traditional medicinal herb, has long been prized for strengthening the immune system. The main ingredients in ginseng, called ginsenosides, have immunomodulatory properties that can boost immunity and increase infection resistance. Supplementing with ginseng has been linked to increased immune cell activity and proliferation, improved synthesis of antibodies, and an increased body's capacity to fight infections.

Furthermore, ginseng has been shown to possess adaptogenic qualities, which support the body's ability to handle stress and preserve homeostasis—a critical condition for the best possible immunological response. Apart from these botanicals, a number of additional herbs and plants, such as astragalus, garlic, and medicinal mushrooms like reishi and shiitake, have also been investigated for their possible immune-boosting properties. These plants include bioactive substances that strengthen the body's defenses, influence immunological responses, and promote immune health in general.

Although there is great promise for improving immune function with botanicals, using them sparingly and with medical advice is essential. Certain botanicals have contraindications for specific medical conditions or may interfere with pharmaceuticals. Additionally, there might be wide variations in the purity and quality of botanical supplements, so it's critical to select reliable companies that follow tight quality control guidelines.

Using botanicals to enhance immunological health is a natural, all-encompassing strategy. Numerous bioactive ingredients found in botanicals, such as ginseng, echinacea, elderberry, and turmeric, can alter immune responses, lessen inflammation, and strengthen the body's defenses against infections. Overall, immune resilience and well-being can be enhanced by including these botanicals in a healthy lifestyle, together with an appropriate diet, enough sleep, frequent exercise, and stress management. Nonetheless, to guarantee safety and effectiveness, it is imperative to approach botanical supplements cautiously and speak with a healthcare provider.

Lifestyle and dietary recommendations for immune health

The significance of preserving a robust immune system has become more apparent in recent times. The body's defense system against dangerous germs, infections, and illnesses is the immune system. Although genetics plays a major role in immune function, dietary and lifestyle choices can also have a big impact. Therefore, promoting general immune health can significantly benefit from forming good habits and including foods that strengthen the immune system in one's diet.

Frequent exercise has been demonstrated to strengthen the immune system and is the cornerstone of a healthy lifestyle. Moderate-intensity exercises like jogging, cycling, or brisk walking should be done for at least thirty minutes most days of the week in order to increase immunity and reduce the risk of chronic illnesses. Improved immune function is a result of exercise's promotion of the body's immune cell circulation, increased antibody synthesis, and decreased inflammatory response.

Getting enough sleep is also essential for keeping your immune system strong. The body goes through critical immunological-supporting activities when you sleep, such as the release of proteins called cytokines, which aid in controlling the immune response. People who experience long-term sleep deprivation are more vulnerable to infections and diseases due to immune system suppression. Adults should strive for 7-9 hours of quality sleep per night to maximize immunological health; children and adolescents may need even more.

Immune system performance and general well-being depend on effective stress management. Extended periods of stress can impair immunity by raising the synthesis of stress hormones like cortisol, which can inhibit immunity. Incorporating stress-relieving practices such as yoga, deep breathing exercises, meditation, or spending time in nature could potentially mitigate the deleterious impact that stress has upon the body's immune system. Furthermore, cultivating relationships with others and upholding a robust support system can offer emotional fortitude, thereby bolstering immune function.

Nutrition is essential for immune function because it provides the building blocks for immunological cells and molecules. An immune system that functions at its best needs a diet that is well-balanced and full of whole grains, fruits, vegetables, lean meats, and healthy fats. Antioxidants, vitamins, minerals, and other bioactive substances that are vital for promoting immune function can be found in these foods. Citrus fruits, broccoli, bell peppers, strawberries, and other vegetables are excellent providers of vitamin C, which is well-known for boosting immunity and lessening the severity and length of colds and other ailments.

Another mineral that is essential for immune function is vitamin D, which also serves to lower inflammation and control immunological responses. Egg yolks, fatty salmon, and fortified dairy products are other excellent food sources of vitamin D, even though sunshine is the best source. By including these foods in the diet, one can promote immune system function and maintain sufficient amounts of vitamin D. Furthermore, zinc—which may be found in beans, nuts, seeds, beef, chicken, oysters, and poultry—is essential for both wound healing and immunological function.

Immune function is supported by probiotics, which are good microorganisms that improve gut health. Trillions of bacteria make up the gut microbiome, which interacts with the immune system and aids in controlling its activity. Consuming probiotic-rich foods like kefir, kimchi, sauerkraut, and yogurt can enhance immune system function and maintain a balanced population of gut bacteria. Additionally, incorporating prebiotic foods such as whole grains, onions, garlic, and bananas into your diet provides the necessary fiber to support the growth of healthy gut flora.

Though it is frequently disregarded, hydration is crucial for immune system health. The body's first line of defense against infections is the mucous membranes in the digestive and respiratory systems, which are kept intact by maintaining adequate hydration. The immune system and general health can be supported by consuming hydrating meals like fruits and vegetables and drinking water throughout the day.

In summary, nutrition and lifestyle choices have a significant impact on immune system support. Through the adoption of health-promoting behaviors, including regular exercise, sufficient rest, stress reduction, and a well-balanced diet high in nutrients that enhance the immune system, people can lower their risk of illness and infection. Choosing preventative measures to boost immune function is crucial to preserving general health and quality of life.

CHAPTER X

Research and Future Directions

Current trends and challenges in herbal antiviral research

In recent years, there has been a sharp increase in interest in and activity surrounding the field of herbal antiviral research, motivated by the pressing need for efficient treatments for viral infections and scientific curiosity. The global community is facing two significant challenges as it attempts to find new antiviral medications derived from natural sources to combat the COVID-19 pandemic. The investigation of traditional medicinal plants that have been utilized for ages in diverse cultures is one of the significant trends in herbal antiviral research. These plants are home to an abundance of bioactive substances that may have antiviral effects; these chemicals could provide valuable leads for future medication research and development.

In addition to traditional expertise, contemporary scientific methods like high-throughput screening and computer modeling are used to identify and describe bioactive compounds from herbal sources. The process of discovery is sped up by researchers' ability to effectively sort through enormous libraries of natural substances thanks to this interdisciplinary methodology. Furthermore, the isolation, purification, and structural elucidation of active ingredients from medicinal plants have been made easier by developments in analytical chemistry and molecular biology, which have also helped to shed light on the mechanisms of action of these constituents against viruses.

In addition, there is growing interest in the supplementary use of traditional herbal therapy in conjunction with contemporary antiviral medications to treat viral infections. Combination therapy with synthetic antiviral medications and plant extracts or phytochemicals has the potential to improve efficacy, lessen side effects, and overcome drug resistance. This all-encompassing method seeks to provide a complete therapeutic approach while acknowledging the intricate relationship between viral pathogenesis and host immunity.

Although there are encouraging tendencies, there are a number of obstacles that prevent advancement in the field of herbal antiviral research. The absence of established procedures for assessing the antiviral efficacy of herbal extracts and chemicals is a significant barrier. The reproducibility and comparability of experimental results can be hampered by variations in extraction techniques, assay systems, and quality control procedures, which can result in inconsistent experimental outcomes. To overcome this problem and guarantee the validity of research findings, standardization initiatives aiming at creating consistent rules and reference materials are crucial.

Furthermore, because natural products have a wide range of chemical compositions and complex plant matrices, it might not be easy to identify and characterize bioactive chemicals from herbal sources. Novel molecule structural elucidation frequently calls for advanced analytical methods like nuclear magnetic resonance spectroscopy and mass spectrometry, which may only be readily available to some researchers. To overcome these technological obstacles and progress in the study of herbal antivirals, chemists, biologists, and pharmacologists must work together.

The inadequate knowledge of the pharmacokinetics and pharmacodynamics of herbal remedies—particularly in relation to antiviral therapy—represents another significant obstacle. The tissue distribution, metabolism, and bioavailability of active substances are some of the factors that affect their safety and efficacy in vivo. Consequently, in order to clarify the absorption, distribution, metabolism, and excretion (ADME) characteristics of herbal products and optimize their dose regimens for clinical usage, thorough pharmacological studies are required.

Regulatory restrictions and intellectual property difficulties further hinder the research and commercialization of herbal antiviral medications. There are obstacles for researchers and producers trying to get their herbal medications approved for the market because of the vast variations in the regulatory structure across nations, which ranges from strict oversight to loose rules. Furthermore, the absence of patent protection for natural goods reduces the incentives for funding the creation of herbal drugs, which could impede innovation in the industry.

In summary, research on herbal antivirals is at a turning point, with both exciting new directions and challenging obstacles to overcome. Combining cutting-edge scientific methods with the investigation of traditional medicinal plants opens up new possibilities for the creation of antiviral solid drugs. However, the conversion of herbal treatments into potent antiviral therapies requires standardizing research methodologies, clarifying pharmacological mechanisms, and navigating regulatory obstacles. Cooperation between researchers, industry players, and regulatory bodies is essential to overcome these obstacles and fully utilize herbal medicine's promise in treating viral infections.

Potential for novel botanical discoveries and formulations

Botanical discoveries and formulations continue to captivate the interest of modern science and medicine. Throughout human civilization, plants have played a vital role in healing, providing nutrition, and inspiring wonderment. Their history is extensive and intricate. We are discovering a wealth of untapped potential as we dive further into the complex field of botany today. Botanical exploration promises new species discovery, the discovery of their medicinal characteristics, and the development of creative therapies to address a wide range of health issues, from the Amazon rainforests to the farthest reaches of the Arctic tundra.

The vast variety of plant species that call our planet home is one of the most fascinating features of botanical inquiry. There are just a few numbers of thoroughly studied and documented plant species worldwide, estimated to number between 300,000 and 500,000. With each species potentially containing unique chemical compounds with undiscovered medical capabilities, this enormous store of biodiversity offers an unrivaled chance for discovery. The potential for new botanical discoveries is almost endless, ranging from obscure plants hiding in the depths of uncharted woods to traditional herbal treatments utilized for generations by indigenous civilizations.

Furthermore, technological developments and improvements in scientific methods have completely changed how we examine and study plant specimens. Botanical research has advanced due to high-throughput screening methods, genetic sequencing, and computer modeling, which have made it possible for scientists to find suitable candidates for additional study with previously unheard-of efficiency. These resources help in the identification of novel plant chemicals as well as the comprehension of their interactions with biological systems, modes of action, and their medical uses.

It is not enough to identify new species or chemicals when it comes to the potential for groundbreaking botanical discoveries. It includes creating novel formulations that take advantage of the medicinal qualities of plants in fresh ways. Modern pharmaceutical techniques are being applied to reinvent and modify traditional herbal medicines, resulting in the development of standardized extracts, encapsulated formulations, and targeted delivery systems. These advancements open the door for innovative therapeutic approaches to a variety of ailments in addition to increasing the efficacy and safety of plant-based medications.

Additionally, because botanical study is multidisciplinary, it encourages cooperation between pharmacology, biochemistry, ethnobotany, and biotechnology. This convergence of expertise makes it easier to explore the possibilities of botanicals holistically, considering ethical considerations, ecological sustainability, and traditional knowledge. Scientists can more adeptly traverse the intricate interactions between plants and human health by combining knowledge from many fields. This allows them to respect cultural heritage and environmental conservation while ensuring that botanical discoveries are transformed into tangible benefits for society.

Botanical discoveries are precious for medicinal purposes and use in agriculture, nutrition, and cosmetics. Compounds produced from plants are being used in agriculture to increase crop yields, strengthen soil, and lessen environmental stresses. Similarly, the nutritional and cosmetic sectors use the rejuvenating, anti-inflammatory, and antioxidant qualities of botanical extracts to create functional foods, skincare products, and dietary supplements that advance health and well-being.

However, coordinated efforts to overcome numerous obstacles are necessary to realize the full potential of botanical discoveries and formulations. Among the many complicated concerns that need to be addressed are the preservation of plant biodiversity, sustainable harvesting methods, intellectual property rights, and regulatory frameworks. Furthermore, there are particular difficulties in bridging the gap between traditional knowledge and scientific confirmation, which calls for polite cooperation with stakeholders and indigenous groups.

In summary, the prospect of new botanical discoveries and formulations is an area that is ready for research and development. Thanks to technological advancements, interdisciplinary cooperation, and a greater comprehension of plant biology, we are on the cusp of a botanical renaissance. We can open up new directions in healthcare, sustainable development, and environmental stewardship by ethically and respectfully utilizing the abundance of nature's pharmacy. This will guarantee a better and more resilient future for coming generations.

Future prospects for integrating herbal medicine into mainstream healthcare

Incorporating herbal medicine into traditional healthcare practices is one viable path to increasing healthcare alternatives and enhancing patient outcomes. Herbal medicine has a long history dating back thousands of years, and it provides a plethora of natural therapeutic options. The advantages of herbal treatments have been more widely acknowledged in recent years, which has prompted more study, legislation, and acceptance in the medical world. Several essential variables point to bright futures for incorporating herbal medicine within traditional healthcare systems.

First, new scientific findings provide insight into the pharmacological workings and effectiveness of many herbal treatments. The biological activities of active components in plant extracts can be identified by scientists using contemporary analytical techniques like mass spectrometry and high-performance liquid chromatography. This scientific confirmation offers a solid basis for incorporating herbal medicines into clinical practice, bridging the gap between conventional wisdom and evidence-based medicine. Furthermore, investigating the synergistic interactions between conventional medications and herbal medicines has the potential to improve treatment outcomes while reducing side effects.

Second, incorporating herbal medicine into conventional practice is propelled by the growing demand for natural and holistic approaches to treatment. As individuals become more health-conscious and search for herbal remedies rather than conventional pharmaceuticals to treat a range of illnesses, herbal medicines are growing in popularity. The increasing demand for integrative medicine clinics and the sales of herbal supplements also show this trend. In order to meet this need, medical professionals are combining herbal medicine into their treatment plans and working with naturopathic and herbalists to provide comprehensive care alternatives.

Thirdly, the incorporation of herbal medicine into conventional healthcare systems is being made more accessible by quality standards and regulatory reforms. Regulatory bodies are realizing that they need to set precise rules for herbal products' efficacy, safety, and quality assurance. The implementation of monographs for herbal compounds and Good Manufacturing Practices (GMP) are two initiatives that aid in ensuring the uniformity and dependability of products. Moreover, the creation of certification programs and professional groups for herbalists and practitioners encourages responsibility and uniformity in the industry. The implementation of regulatory measures fosters confidence between customers and healthcare professionals, hence facilitating the broader recognition and integration of herbal medicine in clinical environments.

Fourth, thanks to technological improvements, patients may now obtain and receive herbal medicine more efficiently. Information regarding herbal treatments, including their applications, dosages, and possible interactions, can be easily accessed through mobile applications and online platforms. Through the use of telemedicine, patients can consult with integrative healthcare professionals and herbalists at a distance, increasing access to herbal medicine in underprivileged areas. Furthermore, advancements in pharmaceutical formulation and delivery technologies, such as standardized extracts and targeted delivery methods, improve the effectiveness and practicality of herbal remedies. These advances in technology enable patients and healthcare practitioners to customize treatment plans to include herbal medication.

Lastly, research and knowledge sharing in the field of herbal medicine are being fueled by partnerships between scientists, traditional healers, and medical professionals. Interdisciplinary research projects unite specialists from several fields to investigate the therapeutic potential of herbal remedies and create evidence-based protocols. Cross-cultural collaborations enable the integration of contemporary scientific methods with the preservation of traditional knowledge systems. Through promoting communication and cooperation, these alliances deepen our knowledge of herbal medicine and aid in its assimilation into mainstream medical practices across the globe.

In summary, there is great potential for the future of incorporating herbal medicine into conventional healthcare due to breakthroughs in science, rising consumer demand, legislative changes, technological advancements, and cooperative partnerships. Herbal medicine will become more and more critical in promoting health, healing, and well-being for people and communities as we investigate the possibilities of herbal medicines and adopt a holistic health approach. Accepting this integration presents chances to improve patient outcomes, increase access to care, and develop a more inclusive, long-lasting healthcare system for coming generations.

CHAPTER XI

Ethnobotanical Perspectives on Viral Defense

Exploration of traditional knowledge and practices of indigenous cultures in combating viral infections using herbal medicine

Indigenous communities possess an abundance of customary wisdom and methods that have been transmitted over many years on the application of herbal medicine for the treatment of viral infections. These civilizations, which are frequently closely linked to the natural world, have created complex systems of herbal treatments that use the therapeutic qualities of plants to treat a range of illnesses, including viral infections. Native American tribes have developed a deep awareness of the medicinal properties of plants through years of observation, research, and cultural transfer. This section explores indigenous societies' traditional knowledge and methods for treating viral infections using herbal medicine, emphasizing the value of maintaining and incorporating these insights into modern healthcare procedures.

For a very long time, indigenous civilizations all over the world have used herbal medicine as their primary treatment for illnesses, including viral infections. Their customary pharmacopeias cover a wide range of plant species, each selected for particular medicinal qualities. Depending on the patient's needs and the type of ailment, these herbal medicines are frequently given as teas, tinctures, poultices, or topical applications. The holistic viewpoint, which emphasizes the significance of reestablishing balance and harmony to attain health and well-being and recognizes the interdependence of body, mind, and spirit, is fundamental to indigenous healing systems.

Native American herbal therapy is notable for its versatility and tenacity in treating newly emergent health issues, such as virus outbreaks. Native American healers possess a profound understanding of local ecosystems and the intricate relationships that exist between plants and their environment. With this information, they may recognize and efficiently apply new herbal cures to fight against diseases that they have just come across. Furthermore, a large number of naturally occurring medicinal herbs have broad-spectrum antiviral qualities that enhance the body's defense against infection by focusing on various phases of viral reproduction. These diverse strategies are in line with integrative medicine's tenets, which mix conventional and traditional treatment practices to get the best possible health outcomes.

Scientific studies have recently started to confirm the effectiveness of traditional herbal medicines in treating viral infections. Numerous bioactive chemicals found in medicinal plants utilized by indigenous tribes have been identified by studies, indicating their potential as sources of new antiviral medicines. In addition, the cooperation of researchers and indigenous healers has made it easier to record and authenticate traditional healing methods, which has opened the door for their incorporation into modern healthcare systems. This multidisciplinary approach advances cultural preservation, builds a deeper appreciation for indigenous knowledge, and improves our understanding of herbal medicine.

Even while traditional herbal therapy has dramatically improved world health, many obstacles and dangers face these techniques. The swift deterioration of the environment, cultural absorption, and financial isolation pose threats to the survival of native medicinal customs, hence risking the loss of priceless wisdom amassed over millennia. Not only does the commercial exploitation of medicinal plants worsen social inequity, but it also jeopardizes efforts to preserve traditional knowledge when it occurs without adequate acknowledgment or benefit-sharing arrangements with indigenous groups.

International, national, and local collaboration is required to address these issues and fully utilize traditional herbal medicine's ability to treat viral infections. This entails putting indigenous peoples' rights and autonomy above their traditional knowledge and genetic resources, developing cooperative relationships based on respect for one another and fair benefit-sharing, and incorporating indigenous healing methods into mainstream healthcare systems. Furthermore, maintaining the sustainability of medicinal plant supplies for future generations depends on conservation initiatives to maintain biodiversity and preserve natural habitats.

In conclusion, research of indigenous cultures' traditional knowledge and methods for utilizing herbal medicine to treat viral infections provides insightful information and practical answers to today's medical problems. Through acknowledging and honoring the knowledge of native healers, we may fully utilize nature's remedy and advance both cultural diversity and health fairness. Adopting an integrated strategy that unites traditional healing techniques and mainstream medicine can potentially create a more sustainable and holistic healthcare paradigm that will benefit present and future generations.

Case studies highlighting the efficacy of ethnobotanical remedies in different regions

Ethnobotanical treatments have been used for a very long time to cure a wide range of illnesses. They are made from native plant species and traditional knowledge. These treatments demonstrate the extraordinary effectiveness of nature's pharmacy while providing fresh perspectives on the complex interrelationship between people and plants. We explore the complex tapestry of ethnobotanical techniques and shed light on their efficacy in addressing health issues through case studies that span many locations.

For millennia, native communities in the Amazon jungle have developed a vast knowledge base of plant-based medicines. One well-known instance is the use of quinine-containing cinchona tree bark to treat malaria. Modern research has confirmed the remedy's efficacy, highlighting the profound wisdom ingrained in conventional medical procedures. Likewise, native Andean people have traditionally used coca leaves—a medicine now known for its vasodilatory qualities—to treat altitude sickness.

Now, let's move to Africa, where a multitude of tribes and cultures continue to employ ethnobotanical treatments. For example, due to their antibacterial qualities, the bitter kola tree's leaves are widely used in Nigeria to cure diseases. In a similar vein, the Rooibos plant is prized in South Africa for its leaves, which are high in antioxidants and can be used as a natural cure for anything from skin disorders to digestive problems.

Ethnobotanical treatments are still widely used in traditional medical systems throughout Asia. The neem tree is highly esteemed in India due to its numerous therapeutic benefits. Neem leaves, seeds, and oil have a wide range of applications in Ayurvedic medicine, including the treatment of diabetes and skin conditions. Similar to this, ginseng, a highly valued herb recognized for its adaptogenic qualities, has been used for millennia in China. Several studies have demonstrated ginseng's potential advantages for enhancing immunity and reducing weariness.

Despite centuries of cultural assimilation, indigenous people in the Americas have managed to maintain their traditional healing techniques. Copal resin is a fragrant tree sap that has deep spiritual and therapeutic value among the Maya of Central America. Copal smoke is used in both therapeutic and ceremonial contexts because it is thought to have cleansing qualities. In a similar vein, specific Indigenous communities in North America have long-valued plants with immune-boosting qualities, like goldenseal and echinacea, as natural substitutes for pharmaceutical drugs.

Even though ethnobotanical traditions include a lot of knowledge, these treatments encounter difficulties in the contemporary environment. Traditional medical knowledge is in danger of being lost due to rapid urbanization, deforestation, and cultural deterioration. Furthermore, commercializing natural resources frequently results in overuse and irresponsible harvesting methods, endangering the precarious equilibrium between people and the environment.

Policymakers, scientists, and indigenous communities must work together to solve these issues and realize the promise of ethnobotanical treatments. These priceless cultural assets can be preserved with the aid of programs that promote community-led healthcare initiatives, encourage sustainable harvesting methods, and archive traditional knowledge.

In conclusion, centuries of traditional use and contemporary scientific validation both attest to the effectiveness of ethnobotanical treatments. We gain an understanding of the profound relationship between humans and plants, which is based on thousands of years of shared history, through case studies from various geographical areas. Adopting the wisdom of ethnobotanical methods can help us better comprehend our place in the natural world and provide us with effective therapeutic modalities while we navigate the challenges of modern healthcare.

CHAPTER XII

Regulatory Landscape and Quality Control of Herbal Products

Overview of regulations governing the production, labeling, and sale of herbal products for viral defense

In the realm of natural health solutions, herbal products have gained significant traction as potential defenses against viral infections. As the world grapples with the complexities of health crises, consumers are increasingly turning to these products in search of preventative measures and immune system support. However, the journey from production to sale of herbal products for viral defense is complex; it is fraught with regulatory considerations to ensure safety, efficacy, and transparency. Across various jurisdictions, stringent regulations govern every aspect of these products, encompassing manufacturing practices, ingredient sourcing, labeling requirements, and marketing claims.

At the heart of regulatory oversight lies the mandate to uphold manufacturing standards that guarantee product safety and quality. Good Manufacturing Practices (GMPs) are applied by organizations like as the US Food and Drug Administration (FDA) and its international counterparts, which are particularly applicable to herbal goods. GMP regulations set forth meticulous guidelines concerning facility cleanliness, equipment maintenance, personnel training, and documentation practices to mitigate contamination risks, adulteration, or misbranding. Compliance with these standards is non-negotiable, as they form the cornerstone of consumer trust and confidence in herbal remedies.

Integral to the production process is the meticulous sourcing and evaluation of herbal ingredients used in these products. Authorities requiring compliance mandate that producers obtain herbs from reliable vendors and submit them to stringent quality assurance procedures. These measures encompass tests for authenticity, purity, potency, and the absence of contaminants such as heavy metals, pesticides, and microbial pathogens. Moreover, adherence to established pharmacopoeial standards, such as the United States Pharmacopeia (USP) or the European Pharmacopoeia (Ph. Eur.), is often mandated to ensure consistency and efficacy across product batches.

As critical as the production process is, the importance of accurate and transparent labeling cannot be overstated. Regulatory bodies require herbal products for viral defense to provide comprehensive information to consumers, including the product name, list of ingredients, dosage instructions, and pertinent warnings or precautions. Furthermore, stringent regulations prohibit manufacturers from making unsubstantiated claims regarding the product's efficacy in preventing or treating viral infections. Claims must be grounded in scientific evidence and devoid of any potential to mislead or deceive consumers.

Navigating the marketing landscape for herbal products poses yet another regulatory challenge. Manufacturers must tread carefully to avoid making therapeutic claims that overstep the bounds of scientific evidence or legality. Advertising materials must be truthful, non-misleading, and compliant with regulations outlined by advertising standards authorities. Neglecting to follow these principles may result in severe penalties, fines, or legal actions that damage a brand's reputation and undermine customer confidence.

Beyond the confines of production and marketing, herbal products for viral defense may be subject to additional regulatory requirements before they can be brought to market. In many jurisdictions, products categorized as medicinal herbs or traditional medicines may necessitate registration or approval akin to pharmaceutical drugs. This entails the submission of comprehensive data pertaining to product formulation, manufacturing processes, quality control measures, and supporting clinical evidence of efficacy and safety.

In conclusion, the journey of herbal products for viral defense from production to sale is fraught with regulatory complexities aimed at safeguarding consumer health and ensuring product integrity. Compliance with Good Manufacturing Practices, stringent ingredient sourcing standards, accurate labeling, and transparent marketing practices are non-negotiable imperatives for manufacturers in this space. By navigating these regulatory frameworks with diligence and integrity, manufacturers can foster consumer trust and confidence in herbal remedies as valuable allies in the ongoing battle against viral infections.

Quality control measures, including authentication, standardization, and testing for purity and potency

Quality control procedures are essential in today's global economy to protect consumer health and preserve confidence across a range of industries, including food, supplements, pharmaceuticals, and more. These procedures, which include standardization, authentication, and potency and purity testing, are the cornerstones that maintain the safety and integrity of the product.

The first line of protection against bogus and inferior goods is authentication. Authentication measures are crucial, especially in the pharmaceutical industry, where counterfeit pharmaceuticals can have dire repercussions.

Manufacturers can confirm the validity of their products by precisely identifying active components and excipients through the use of technologies like spectroscopy and chromatography. Businesses may make sure that their drugs have the required ingredients in the right amounts by comparing chromatographic profiles or spectral signatures to reference standards. In addition to shielding consumers from potentially dangerous materials, this preserves the good name of accredited producers.

Standardization ensures consistency and effectiveness by creating uniformity in products, which is a complement to authenticity. The permissible range of parameters within the pharmaceutical industry, including composition, purity, and strength, is determined by compliance with pharmacopeial standards. These standards give producers precise instructions so they can make drugs that satisfy legal requirements and have consistent therapeutic effects. In the food business, standardization is equally crucial since it guarantees uniformity in the sensory qualities, nutritional makeup, and labeling details. Food businesses can improve consumer safety and confidence while also making regulatory agency compliance easier by following standard operating procedures.

The last stage of quality control involves testing for potency and purity, which guarantees that goods fulfill predetermined criteria. Strict analytical methods are used in the pharmaceutical industry to ensure that active substances are potent and that no contaminants are present. For example, high-performance liquid chromatography (HPLC) is frequently used to measure contaminants with remarkable sensitivity, guaranteeing that pharmaceuticals adhere to strict regulatory standards. Similar to this, potency testing confirms the concentration of bioactive substances in dietary supplements, guaranteeing their efficacy and accuracy on labels. Additionally, by identifying dangerous infections and verifying adherence to microbiological limitations, microbial testing is essential to guarantee the safety of products. Both the health of consumers and the manufacturers' reputations depend on these testing protocols.

Strict laws and global norms regulate the application of quality control methods, highlighting their significance in preserving public health. These standards are established and enforced in large part by regulatory bodies like the European Medicines Agency (EMA) in Europe and the Food and Drug Administration (FDA) in the United States. These organizations make sure that manufacturers follow best practices and create high-quality, safe products by establishing explicit criteria and carrying out inspections. International cooperation and harmonization initiatives also support worldwide uniformity in quality control standards and expedite regulatory procedures.

Although conventional methods of quality control have demonstrated efficacy, technological developments present novel prospects for augmenting product safety and integrity. Artificial intelligence (AI) and blockchain are two emerging technologies that have the potential to transform quality control procedures completely. Supply chains may be made transparent and traceable thanks to blockchain technology's decentralized and unchangeable ledger system. Blockchain enables participants to confirm the legitimacy and integrity of goods at every stage of manufacturing and distribution by keeping track of all transactions and interactions along the supply chain. Similar to this, producers may detect any deviations and proactively reduce risks by using AI algorithms to speed up data processing and pattern recognition. With the use of these technologies, quality control procedures have become much more effective and efficient, producing goods that are safer and more dependable for customers.

Implementing quality control techniques still needs to be improved despite its many advantages. For both manufacturers and regulatory authorities, the growth of sophisticated counterfeit methods and the complexity of global supply networks pose constant hurdles. Collaboration amongst stakeholders, such as industry partners, regulators, and technology suppliers, is necessary to address these difficulties. Stakeholders can create more effective plans for thwarting fake and inferior goods by exchanging knowledge and best practices. In addition, creating and sustaining efficient quality control systems requires investments in infrastructure and worker training.

To sum up, quality control procedures such as authentication, standardization, and potency and purity testing are critical for guaranteeing product integrity and safety in a variety of businesses. Manufacturers can preserve consumer health and product trust by putting in place strict quality control procedures and following legal requirements. Furthermore, technological developments present fresh chances to raise the efficacy and efficiency of quality control procedures, bolstering their significance in maintaining public health. We will constantly need to innovate and work together to sustain the highest standards of quality and safety as we take on new challenges in the global economy.

CHAPTER XIII

Safety and Side Effects of Herbal Antivirals

Discussion on the safety profile of herbal remedies, including potential adverse effects and interactions with medications

With a long history dating back hundreds of years, herbal treatments provide a safe, natural solution to conventional medication for a wide range of medical issues. But as these treatments get more and more well- liked, it becomes more crucial to comprehend their safety profile, including any potential side effects and drug interactions. Although many herbs have medicinal properties, they have hazards that need to be carefully considered and closely observed.

The possibility of adverse effects is one of the main worries about herbal medicines. In contrast to pharmaceutical drugs, herbal medications may contain different amounts of active ingredients and sometimes lack established dosing. Individual responses may vary due to this variability, from minor discomfort to serious negative consequences. For instance, when taken in high doses or in combination with other medications that alter serotonin levels, some herbs, like St. John's Wort, which is frequently used for mood disorders like depression, have been linked to adverse effects like gastrointestinal distress, allergic reactions, and even serotonin syndrome.

Furthermore, there's a chance that certain herbal medicines will interact negatively or less effectively with over-the-counter or prescription drugs. Numerous factors, such as modifications in drug metabolism, pharmacokinetics, or pharmacodynamics, may give rise to these interactions. Research has demonstrated, for example, that supplements containing garlic, which are well-liked for their possible cardiovascular advantages, can inhibit the activity of cytochrome P450 enzymes, which are crucial for the metabolism of several medications. This could result in higher blood levels of warfarin and antiplatelet medications, which increase the risk of bleeding.

Furthermore, bioactive substances included in herbal medicines have the potential to mimic or obstruct the effects of prescription medications, resulting in unexpected side effects.For example, the terpenoids and flavonoids in ginkgo biloba, a herb that is frequently used to improve cognitive function, may inhibit platelet aggregation and increase bleeding risk, particularly when combined with anticoagulant medications such as aspirin or warfarin. Comparably, using herbal supplements like echinacea, which is praised for strengthening the immune system, may interact with how some medications are metabolized, decreasing their efficacy or raising the risk of toxicity.

Herbal treatments are not subject to the same stringent regulatory scrutiny as pharmaceutical drugs, which results in gaps in quality control and safety data despite these possible concerns. Many herbal items are sold as dietary supplements, enabling producers to avoid going through the rigorous approval and testing procedures needed for pharmaceuticals. Consequently, there can be wide variations in the potency, purity, and safety of herbal treatments among different brands and products, which makes it difficult for consumers and healthcare professionals to make wise choices.

Healthcare professionals and patients need to have honest conversations about the use of herbal treatments in order to reduce the hazards involved. In order to enable thorough medication management and risk assessment, patients should be urged to reveal all herbal supplements they are taking in addition to any prescription or over- the-counter medications. To assist patients in making educated decisions, healthcare providers can offer evidence-based information regarding the efficacy and safety of particular herbal medicines as well as possible interactions with prescription drugs.

Healthcare professionals should also be on the lookout for any indications of adverse effects or drug interactions in patients who use herbal treatments, especially if they have complicated medical histories or are taking several prescriptions. For those who are more susceptible to herb-drug interactions, routine monitoring of laboratory measures, such as coagulation studies or liver function tests, may be necessary. Furthermore, healthcare providers must remain current on the latest research and regulatory updates pertaining to herbal products to guarantee that patients receive safe and efficient care.

In summary, although herbal medicines have the potential to be therapeutically beneficial, there are inherent dangers associated with them, such as negative interactions with drugs and side effects. Healthcare professionals are essential in informing patients about the safety profile of herbal treatments and keeping an eye out for any possible drug interactions or side effects. Healthcare providers can assist patients in navigating the complicated world of herbal medicine while maintaining their safety and well-being by encouraging open communication and teamwork.

Guidance on mitigating risks and ensuring safe usage through proper dosage and monitoring

Navigating the difficulties of pharmaceutical consumption is a critical undertaking in the field of healthcare. A comprehensive strategy is needed to ensure the safe administration of drugs, with careful monitoring and appropriate dosage serving as essential cornerstones in reducing risks and improving patient outcomes. The importance of monitoring and dose guidelines for ensuring patient safety and advancing efficient medication administration is discussed in this section.

The correct dosage, individualized for each patient's needs, must be prescribed and administered. This is the foundation of safe pharmaceutical use. While determining the proper dosage for a specific prescription, healthcare providers must carefully consider a number of criteria, including age, weight, renal and hepatic function, and potential drug interactions. Precise dosing is essential for optimizing the advantages of drug therapy while lowering the dangers involved. Noncompliance with suggested dosage parameters might result in adverse effects like toxicity or therapeutic ineffectiveness. It is crucial to provide patients with precise dosing recommendations so they can actively participate in their care and carefully follow recommended schedules.

Monitoring patients' responses to drug therapy on a continuous basis is equally essential in order to identify and swiftly address any new problems. The efficacy and safety of the recommended pharmaceutical regimen can be assessed by healthcare professionals through routine evaluations of clinical data, laboratory results, and adverse drug reactions. Early detection of possible issues such as pharmaceutical toxicity, insufficient therapeutic response, or drug interactions enables prompt intervention and if needed, modification of the treatment strategy. Additionally, patient education is essential for encouraging self-monitoring and enabling people to identify and promptly report any adverse effects or changes in their condition.

Technological developments in the last several years have greatly improved the ability of medical practitioners to monitor and control pharmaceutical dosage.

The use of computerized physician order entry (CPOE) systems and electronic health records (EHRs) during the prescription and administration of medication reduces medication safety and mistake rates. Clinical decision support systems (CDSS) facilitate adherence to evidence-based prescribing procedures and improve patient safety by giving doctors real-time alerts and reminders. Furthermore, cutting-edge approaches to remote monitoring and patient involvement are provided via telehealth platforms and smartphone apps, which enable ongoing monitoring of medication adherence and health conditions outside of conventional healthcare settings.

To ensure thorough and well-coordinated drug administration, healthcare personnel must collaborate across interdisciplinary fields. Together, pharmacists, doctors, nurses, and other allied health specialists must create customized treatment programs that put patient safety first and maximize therapeutic results. Pharmacists can participate more actively in medication optimization initiatives by conducting complete medication evaluations and offering patients helpful education and assistance through collaborative practice models like medication therapy management (MTM) services. Healthcare professionals may guarantee that patients receive comprehensive care that addresses their specific drug needs and reduces the likelihood of adverse events by encouraging communication and collaboration throughout healthcare professions.

In summary, recommendations for risk reduction and safe pharmaceutical use through appropriate dosage and monitoring are critical for improving patient outcomes and elevating the standard of healthcare as a whole. Healthcare providers can prioritize patient safety and well-being while managing medication safely by following evidence-based prescribing practices, performing routine monitoring assessments, utilizing technological advancements, and encouraging interdisciplinary collaboration. A thorough approach to drug safety must include giving patients the knowledge and resources they need to make informed decisions about their care as well as enabling them to engage in it actively. In the end, healthcare workers can maintain the most excellent standards of care and help all patients have better health outcomes by adhering to these principles.

CHAPTER XIV

Herbal Medicine in Special Populations

Considerations for using herbal remedies in vulnerable populations such as children, elderly individuals, pregnant women, and those with underlying health conditions

For millennia, people have used herbal treatments as a natural substitute for traditional medication to treat a range of health issues. However, in order to guarantee safety and effectiveness, a number of important factors must be taken into account when considering their use in vulnerable groups, such as children, the elderly, pregnant women, and people with underlying medical disorders.

To begin with, children are a particular group of people who develop physiological systems. Compared to adults, their bodies might respond to herbal medicines differently, which could result in unanticipated side effects or interactions. It is crucial to take dosage into account because children may need lower doses in relation to their body weight in order to prevent adverse side effects. Furthermore, because some herbs have the ability to impede growth and development or worsen pre-existing illnesses, they might not be appropriate for kids. Therefore, it is essential to speak with a doctor or other experienced healthcare provider before giving children herbal medications.

In a similar vein, older adults may have various chronic medical issues and may be taking multiple drugs at once. Prescription medications and herbal treatments may interact negatively or lessen the effectiveness of both treatments. Furthermore, the absorption, distribution, metabolism, and excretion of herbal substances might be impacted by age-related changes in metabolism and organ function, which calls for careful evaluation of dosage adjustments and potential dangers. In order to guarantee the safe incorporation of herbal remedies into the treatment regimen of older patients, healthcare providers must be involved in the decision-making process.

Another susceptible group to whom the use of herbal treatments should be approached with caution is pregnant women. The safety of several herbs during pregnancy has not been thoroughly investigated, and some may increase the risk of miscarriage, early labor, or problems in development. There may be conflicting information about the safety of using common herbs like ginger and chamomile during pregnancy. Therefore, before utilizing herbal treatments to treat pregnancy-related symptoms or medical disorders, pregnant women should use caution and speak with obstetricians or midwives.

Moreover, caution should be exercised while contemplating herbal medicines by those with underlying medical illnesses, such as diabetes, hypertension, or autoimmune disorders. Certain herbs have the potential to worsen underlying medical disorders or interfere with drugs used to treat these conditions. Herbs such as garlic and ginseng, for example, have the potential to conflict with anticoagulant drugs, increasing the risk of bleeding in people with heart conditions. Moreover, there may be significant differences in the quality and purity of herbal products, increasing the risk of infection or adulteration, particularly in vulnerable populations with compromised immune systems or impaired detoxification procedures.

Cultural and socioeconomic variables may impact the accessibility and utilization of herbal treatments in disadvantaged communities, aside from potential interactions with drugs and safety issues. People who have limited access to standard medicine or healthcare facilities may turn to alternative medicines, such as herbal cures, which are only sometimes safe or supported by evidence. Promoting informed decision-making about the use of herbal treatments in vulnerable groups requires education and awareness initiatives aimed at the general public as well as healthcare providers.

In summary, even though herbal treatments have a lot of potential therapeutic applications, using them in susceptible groups, including young children, the elderly, pregnant women, and people with underlying medical issues, needs careful evaluation of the advantages and disadvantages. In order to ensure the safe and successful integration of herbal medicines into patient care plans, cooperation between healthcare providers, patients, and practitioners of herbal medicine is essential. Through adherence to evidence-based methods and open communication, we can minimize possible harm in vulnerable populations while optimizing the use of herbal treatments.

Adaptations of herbal protocols and dosage adjustments for different age groups and health statuses

With its roots in antiquity and support from contemporary science, herbal medicine provides a wide range of treatments that may be customized to meet the specific requirements of people of different ages and health conditions. The more we learn about the nuances of herbal protocols and dosage modifications, the more obvious it is that there is no one-size-fits-all solution to the complex issues surrounding human health. Instead, in order to maximize therapeutic results and guarantee patient safety, herbalists and medical professionals need to take into account variables, including age, underlying medical disorders, metabolic variations, and possible interactions with prescription drugs.

It is essential to acknowledge that there are substantial differences in the physiological traits and health requirements of newborns, children, adults, and older people while investigating the modifications of herbal regimens for various age groups. Herbal treatments should be given with extreme caution to infants and young children due to their fragile and developing bodies. Doses need to be carefully determined based on weight and age, and any concurrent drugs or herbs should be taken into account for potential interactions.

Furthermore, some herbs might not be appropriate for pediatric patients because of their strength or potential for side effects. As a result, herbal formulations for this age range frequently contain mild herbs that have a long history of being safe when given to kids in the correct forms, including glycerites or diluted tinctures.

As we move on to adulthood, herbal treatments can become more standardized, but modifications are still required to consider individual health statuses and metabolic variations. Adults can present with a variety of problems, ranging from acute illnesses to chronic disorders, each of which needs a customized herbal remedy plan. For instance, those with liver or kidney damage might need to choose herbs with nephroprotective or hepatoprotective qualities, or their dosages might need to be adjusted. In a similar vein, people with allergies or sensitivities should stay away from herbs that are known to cause adverse reactions. Still, people who have long-term health issues like diabetes or hypertension could benefit from herbs that aid with managing their particular issues.

Herbal medicine must take special care of elderly patients due to age-related metabolism and organ function changes. Due to the body's deteriorating ability to absorb and eliminate chemicals, older persons may be more susceptible to the effects of herbs and medications. As a result, dosage modifications are frequently required to guarantee therapeutic efficacy and avoid unpleasant reactions. Furthermore, as age-related digestive problems may impair the bioavailability of herbal ingredients, herbal formulations for older people should be reduced to improve digestion and absorption. Furthermore, as older people are more likely to be taking many prescriptions at once, thought should be given to possible herb-drug interactions.

Herbal protocol modifications go beyond age categories, including various health conditions and lifestyle choices. Immuno-supportive herbs can help people with weakened immune systems—such as those receiving chemotherapy or living with HIV/AIDS—by boosting their body's ability to fight off infections. Herbs that enhance general vitality, lessen inflammation, and aid in muscle rehabilitation may be necessary for athletes and people with busy lifestyles. Herbs used by expectant or nursing mothers must be carefully chosen to prevent harm to the growing fetus or baby; some herbs should not be used because they may cause uterine contractions or upset the balance of hormones.

Modifications in dosage are essential for maximizing the safety and effectiveness of herbal remedies across a range of demographics. When determining the proper dosages, factors including body weight, metabolic rate, and personal tolerance levels must be considered. Particularly for pediatric dosages, exact computation is necessary to prevent under- or overdose; liquid herbal extracts are frequently chosen because of their convenient administration and precise dosing capabilities. Adult dosages may differ according to the severity of the ailment being treated and the herbal preparation's potency; modifications are made as necessary to maximize therapeutic benefits and reduce the possibility of adverse effects.

Furthermore, dosage modifications and treatment results may be impacted by the mode of administration. Although the most popular way to administer herbal remedies is by mouth, there are times when topical treatments, inhalation, or suppositories are more appropriate. The need to customize the route of administration to individual preferences and health needs is underscored by the fact that each route has unique concerns about dosage, absorption rates, and potential side effects.

In summary, critical components of individualized herbal treatment include modifying dosages and adapting herbal procedures for various age groups and health conditions. Herbalists and other healthcare professionals can maximize therapeutic benefits while lowering the possibility of side effects by considering each patient's particular needs and traits. Herbal medicine is developing as a valuable complement to existing healthcare methods based on a blend of scientific understanding, clinical experience, and traditional wisdom. It provides a safe and efficient means of fostering overall health.

CHAPTER XV

Cultivation, Sustainability, and Conservation of Medicinal Plants

Importance of sustainable practices in harvesting and cultivating medicinal plants for viral defense

The importance of medicinal plants in fending off viral dangers has increasingly come to light in the aftermath of the worldwide health crisis. The collection and production of these plants must follow sustainable procedures as humanity confronts more complex health issues. In this particular context, the significance of sustainability is immense, as it guarantees the conservation of biodiversity, upholds the equilibrium of ecosystems, and protects the effectiveness of medical resources for the next generations. Sustainable harvesting methods take into account the effects on the environment, show respect for local people and traditional knowledge, and follow moral standards.

First, knowing the biological dynamics of medicinal plants' native environments is essential to sustainable medicinal plant harvesting. Overuse and careless harvesting can cause habitat degradation, biodiversity loss, and even the extinction of entire plant species. We may reduce these threats and guarantee the long-term survival of medicinal plant populations by using sustainable harvesting practices, including selective harvesting, site rotation, and consideration for seasonal fluctuations in plant growth. Furthermore, sustainable harvesting methods support ecosystem conservation by protecting important habitats for a variety of flora and fauna that are essential to the functioning of ecosystems.

Second, there are several advantages to growing medicinal plants using sustainable farming methods. Plant development can be optimized in a controlled setting through cultivation, which lessens the strain on wild populations. Sustainable farming techniques that emphasize soil health reduce chemical inputs, and foster biodiversity include organic, permaculture, and agroforestry. Adding medicinal plants to agroecosystems not only makes the ecosystem more resilient but also opens up new markets for farmers, especially in rural areas where access to healthcare may be limited.

Furthermore, sustainable farming and harvesting methods recognize the inextricable connection between environmental and human health. Viral infections are a prime example of how ecosystems and human societies are intertwined. We strengthen our resistance to newly developing infectious diseases, particularly viral risks, by protecting natural habitats and biodiversity. Traditional healers have been using the antiviral properties of several therapeutic herbs for millennia. The sustainable gathering and nurturing of these priceless resources aids the development of innovative antiviral therapies and vaccines.

Furthermore, sustainable methods support cultural preservation and social fairness. Indigenous groups and traditional healers frequently possess invaluable knowledge regarding the therapeutic qualities of plants and their long-term applications. Sustainable practices must include them in decision-making processes, respect their rights, and acknowledge their expertise. We promote social justice and fortify our collective resistance to health crises by strengthening local communities and protecting indigenous knowledge systems.

In summary, the importance of sustainable practices in the cultivation and collection of medicinal plants for the purpose of protecting against viruses cannot be overstated. By implementing sustainable practices, we can protect ecosystems, conserve biodiversity, improve human health, and advance social justice. Sustainable practices must continue to be at the forefront of our efforts to maximize the potential of medicinal plants in countering viral threats as we traverse the difficulties of the twenty-first century. We can only create a future for future generations that is healthier and more robust by taking proper care of nature's resources.

Initiatives for conserving biodiversity, promoting ethical wildcrafting, and supporting local communities

In the face of escalating environmental challenges, initiatives targeting the conservation of biodiversity, promoting ethical wildcrafting practices, and supporting local communities have emerged as critical strategies for fostering sustainable development and safeguarding our planet's ecological integrity. Biodiversity, encompassing the richness and variety of life forms on Earth, lies at the heart of ecosystem health and resilience. Protecting species and their habitats from hazards like pollution, climate change, and habitat degradation is necessary to preserve biodiversity. One of the most prominent initiatives for biodiversity conservation involves the establishment and management of protected areas. These areas serve as havens for wildlife, preserving critical habitats and ecological processes. Moreover, they offer opportunities for scientific research, environmental education, and eco-tourism, thereby generating awareness and support for conservation efforts.

Ethical wildcrafting, the sustainable harvesting of wild plants and other natural resources, has gained traction to promote biodiversity conservation while meeting human needs. Wildcrafting encompasses various practices, including gathering medicinal herbs, collecting wild edibles, and harvesting materials for crafts and cultural purposes. To ensure the long-term viability of wildcrafting activities, ethical guidelines and harvesting protocols are essential. These guidelines prioritize sustainable harvesting methods, such as selective harvesting, which involves gathering only a portion of the available plant material to allow for natural regeneration. Furthermore, wildcrafters are encouraged to respect seasonal and spatial distribution patterns, minimize habitat disturbance, and obtain appropriate permits or permissions when harvesting from protected areas or private lands.

Local communities, particularly indigenous and traditional societies, play a pivotal role in biodiversity conservation and sustainable resource management. These communities often possess invaluable knowledge about local ecosystems, including traditional land-use practices, ecological indicators, and biodiversity hotspots. Engaging with local communities as partners in conservation efforts enhances conservation strategies' effectiveness and promotes social equity and cultural diversity.

Collaborative approaches that integrate traditional ecological knowledge with scientific research can lead to innovative conservation solutions tailored to local contexts. Furthermore, empowering local communities through capacity-building initiatives, income-generating projects, and equitable benefit-sharing mechanisms strengthens their resilience and fosters a sense of ownership and stewardship over natural resources.

Supporting local economies and livelihoods is essential for achieving sustainable development goals and reducing pressure on natural ecosystems. Conservation initiatives that provide alternative income opportunities to local communities can help alleviate poverty and dependence on unsustainable resource extraction. For example, eco-tourism initiatives that offer guided nature tours, homestays, and cultural experiences not only generate revenue for local communities but also raise awareness about the value of biodiversity and the importance of conservation. Similarly, agroforestry projects that promote the cultivation of native species alongside food crops can enhance ecosystem resilience, improve soil fertility, and diversify income sources for rural farmers.

In conclusion, initiatives focused on conserving biodiversity, promoting ethical wildcrafting practices, and supporting local communities are indispensable for addressing the interconnected challenges of environmental degradation, species loss, and socio-economic inequality. Our world and its inhabitants may have a more robust and egalitarian future if we prioritize ecosystem conservation, adopt sustainable resource management techniques, and encourage community empowerment. Collaboration among governments, non-governmental organizations, indigenous peoples, local communities, and other stakeholders is crucial for scaling up these initiatives and achieving meaningful conservation outcomes on a global scale. Together, we can work towards a world where biodiversity thrives, ecosystems flourish, and communities thrive in harmony with nature.

CHAPTER XVI

Herbal Medicine and Viral Resistance

Examination of the phenomenon of viral resistance to herbal treatments and strategies to minimize resistance development

The development of herbal treatment-resistant viruses poses a severe obstacle to the fight against infectious diseases. Although herbal therapies have been utilized for a long time due to their medicinal capabilities, over time, these treatments may become less effective due to resistance caused by the fast development of viruses. Understanding the mechanisms driving viral resistance and putting strategies in place to reduce its development are necessary to maintain the efficacy of herbal medications.

Viral Opposition to Herbal Remedies. Numerous reasons frequently lead to the development of viral resistance to natural remedies. First of all, viruses can swiftly adapt to environmental stresses, such as exposure to herbal components, due to their fast rate of mutation. Furthermore, viruses can develop resistance by means of processes such as modification of the viral target sites or overexpression of efflux pumps, which remove herbal substances from cells that are infected. Additionally, improper or excessive use of herbal medicines can hasten the emergence of resistance since insufficient dosages may not be enough to stop viral replication, allowing resistant strains to survive and proliferate.

Techniques to Reduce the Development of Resistance. Several tactics can be used to address the problem of viral resistance to natural remedies. The first step in making the most out of using herbal treatments is to make sure that the correct dosage and administration procedures are followed. This entails refraining from self-medication without supervision and seeking advice from licensed healthcare providers regarding the proper application of herbal remedies. Additionally, by lessening the selective pressure on virus populations, switching between herbal medicines with various mechanisms of action can help prevent the establishment of resistance.

Moreover, combining herbal remedies with traditional antiviral medications can improve their effectiveness and lower the chance that resistance will grow. Herbal and synthetic medication interactions work synergistically to overcome resistance mechanisms and enhance therapeutic effects. Furthermore, in agricultural contexts where virus resistance can have disastrous effects on crop output, adding herbal medicines into integrated pest management systems might help preserve their effectiveness.

Investing in research to comprehend the mechanisms of viral resistance to herbal medicines is crucial, in addition to optimizing treatment options. Researchers can create new herbal compounds with improved potency against resistant viruses and find possible targets for drug development by clarifying the molecular mechanisms involved in resistance development.

Reducing the establishment of resistance also requires public education and awareness campaigns. We can encourage a culture of informed decision-making and treatment adherence by teaching patients, healthcare professionals, and the general public about the significance of using herbal medicines responsibly and the dangers of resistance.

In conclusion, a significant obstacle in the fight against infectious diseases is the phenomenon of viral resistance to natural remedies. However, we can maintain the effectiveness of herbal medicines and guarantee their continuous usefulness in treating viral infections by comprehending the mechanisms driving resistance development and putting policies in place to avoid its occurrence. By working together, researchers, medical professionals, and legislators may create comprehensive strategies to deal with this urgent problem and protect public health.

Rotation of herbal remedies, combination therapies, and alternative approaches to overcome resistance

The conventional emphasis on monotherapies has frequently proven ineffective in the never-ending fight against resistance, resulting in the creation of resilient infections and malignancies that are resistant to therapy. However, a paradigm shift is in progress as a result of the growing awareness of the many advantages provided by rotating approaches that use herbal medicines. Herbal rotation, a long-standing technique based on the tenets of ancient medical systems, alternates between various plant preparations to prevent infections or cancerous cells from adapting. This strategy makes sense because different plants have different biochemical compositions and contain different kinds of phytochemicals with different modes of action. It is less likely for resistance to develop when the herbal composition is regularly altered, providing a long-term answer to treatment problems. Moreover, there is great potential for overcoming resistance when combining herbal medicines with conventional therapies. By carefully combining botanical components with pharmaceutical treatments, one can maximize their synergistic interactions and reduce the likelihood of resistance emerging, hence increasing therapeutic efficacy. By utilizing the complimentary modes of action, this integrative approach addresses the inherent limits of monotherapy and improves therapeutic outcomes. Furthermore, complementary and alternative therapies like Ayurveda, TCM, and acupuncture provide new paths through resistance. These all-encompassing methods place a high priority on the body's natural defenses and resilience against harmful or malignant threats—essentially, restoring homeostasis inside the body. Alternative therapies not only reduce the likelihood of resistance but also create an atmosphere that is best suited for the most beneficial therapeutic results by addressing underlying imbalances and fostering holistic well-being.

Using a multimodal approach, the rotation of herbal treatments is a dynamic technique that leverages the intrinsic diversity of botanicals to prevent the emergence of resistance. Herbal rotation disturbs adaptive systems by exposing infections or cancer cells to novel biochemical elements on a constant basis, in contrast to traditional monotherapies that provide selective pressure. This proactive strategy not only prevents resistance from developing but also fosters therapeutic synergy, which increases the effectiveness of treatment. Furthermore, because herbal medicines are so adaptable, customized interventions can be made to meet the specific requirements and reactions of each patient. Clinicians can minimize the danger of developing resistance while optimizing therapeutic effects by implementing customized herbal rotation programs.

Simultaneously, the combination of herbal treatments and traditional therapies provides a tactical method to address resistance on several fronts. Synergistic interactions between botanical and synthetic drugs can be used to overcome resistance mechanisms and improve treatment efficacy. By addressing the drawbacks of monotherapy and broadening therapeutic options, this integrated strategy extends the efficacy of treatment plans. Combination therapy also reduces side effects and allows for a decrease in dose, which enhances patient tolerance and treatment compliance.

Alternative methods that provide comprehensive tactics to strengthen immunity and resilience against resistance include acupuncture, Ayurveda, and TCM. These traditional therapeutic techniques place a high priority on the body's ability to regain equilibrium, treating underlying imbalances that lead to the appearance of resistance. Alternative therapies fortify the body's natural defense mechanisms, making it less vulnerable to pathogenic or malignant threats by fostering harmony between mind, body, and spirit. Furthermore, by allowing patients to engage in their recovery process actively, these holistic methods promote patients' sense of empowerment and self-efficacy.

To sum up, using combination therapies, rotating herbal cures, and using alternative methods are creative ways to address resistance in healthcare. Clinicians can maximize treatment outcomes while navigating the complexity of resistance by utilizing the combined power of different approaches. The secret to transforming patient care and overcoming therapeutic obstacles in the twenty-first century lies in adopting holistic and integrative approaches as we continue to untangle the complexities of resistance mechanisms.

CHAPTER XVII

Case Studies and Clinical Applications

Real-life case studies illustrating the application of herbal medicine in the management and treatment of viral infections

In recent years, there has been a growing interest in the use of herbal therapy in the management and treatment of viral infections. Herbal treatments have been used for centuries in many traditional medical systems around the world. They are made from plants and other natural sources. Today, herbal therapy is becoming more and more recognized as a potential adjunct to traditional antiviral medications due to advances in scientific study and a deeper understanding of the therapeutic characteristics of plants. Case studies from real-world situations provide strong proof of the effectiveness and safety of herbal treatments in the treatment of viral infections.

Sambucus nigra Elderberries for the Treatment of Influenza The use of elderberry extract to treat influenza is one noteworthy case study. Because of its ability to strengthen the immune system, elderberry, which is produced from the fruit of the Sambucus nigra plant, has long been used in traditional medicine. Researchers examined the effectiveness of elderberry syrup in the treatment of influenza symptoms in a randomized controlled experiment that was published in the Journal of International Medical Research. Comparing the elderberry extract group to the placebo group, the study revealed that the former significantly improved in terms of symptoms, including fever, headache, and nasal congestion. The potential of elderberry as a home treatment for managing influenza is demonstrated by this case study.

Glycyrrhiza glabra, Licorice, and the Herpes Simplex Virus

The antiviral efficacy of licorice root extract against the herpes simplex virus (HSV) is another noteworthy case study. The Glycyrrhiza glabra plant's root is used to make licorice, which is a plant root that contains bioactive substances with antiviral solid qualities. A study showing the inhibitory effects of licorice extract on HSV replication in vitro was reported in the Journal of Ethnopharmacology. In addition, topical licorice cream treatment dramatically decreased the length and severity of herpes lesions in a clinical trial of patients with recurrent HSV infections. The potential of licorice as a topical therapy for HSV infections is highlighted by this case study.

The Management of HIV/AIDS Using Astragalus

(Astragalus membranaceus) Due to its immunomodulatory properties, astragalus, a herbaceous plant native to China, has long been utilized in Chinese medicine. A case study published in the Journal of Alternative and Complementary Medicine demonstrated the efficacy of astragalus supplements in managing HIV/AIDS. The study drew from real-life experiences to illustrate its findings. The case study was based on actual experiences. The research monitored individuals with HIV who were prescribed astragalus extract in addition to their usual antiretroviral therapy. Astragalus supplementation improved CD4 cell counts and suppressed viral loads, according to the results, pointing to a possible role for the supplement in improving immune function and lowering viral replication in HIV/AIDS patients. This case study demonstrates the potentially beneficial additional effects of astragalus in the treatment of HIV and other viral diseases.

Allium sativum Garlic as a Protective Agent Against Respiratory Viral Illnesses Garlic is well known for strengthening the immune system and having antibacterial properties; it has also been investigated as a potential therapy for viral respiratory infections. A real-world case study that was published in the British Journal of Biomedical Science looked at the effectiveness of supplementing with Garlic to prevent and lessen common cold symptoms. Compared to the placebo group, those who took Garlic extract had fewer cold episodes and milder symptoms. Moreover, investigations conducted in vitro have shown that garlic components have antiviral effects against respiratory viruses like rhinovirus and influenza. The therapeutic potential of Garlic as a home treatment for respiratory viral infections is highlighted by this case study.

In conclusion. Case studies from real life offer essential insights into how herbal medicine can be used to manage and treat viral infections. These case studies highlight the various antiviral qualities of herbal treatments, ranging from elderberry for influenza to licorice for herpes simplex virus and from astragalus for HIV/AIDS to Garlic for respiratory viral infections. Herbal medicine has the potential to be an adjunct to traditional antiviral treatments, providing safer and more readily available choices for patients globally, even though additional study is required to clarify the mechanisms of action and enhance therapy procedures.

Clinical trials and observational studies evaluating the efficacy of herbal interventions

In the pursuit of determining the effectiveness of herbal therapies, clinical trials, and observational research are essential instruments. These approaches offer strict standards for assessing the efficacy, safety, and practical implications of herbal treatments, which have been used for centuries in many cultures. Clinical trials, which are distinguished by their randomized, double-masked designs, provide controlled settings in which the effectiveness of herbal remedies can be methodically evaluated in comparison to established treatments or placebos. Nevertheless, there are particular difficulties in carrying out clinical trials for herbal remedies, such as standardizing items and dosages to guarantee uniformity and repeatability. However, these studies continue to be essential in developing evidence-based guidelines for herbal remedies, especially when it comes to common medical diseases for which traditional treatments could prove ineffective.

Conversely, observational studies provide further information about the efficacy and security of herbal therapies in real-world contexts. Through the observation of individuals who self-administer herbal treatments in their daily lives, researchers can obtain essential insights about treatment patterns, long-term benefits, and possible side effects. Even while observational studies don't have the same experimental control as clinical trials, they offer a comprehensive picture of herbal use across a range of demographics, illuminating the subtle differences in the efficacy of herbal interventions outside of controlled environments. Moreover, observational studies play a crucial role in pointing out patterns and correlations that could need more study in clinical trials, helping to shape focused research goals.

Numerous herbal remedies have been examined in clinical trials and observational research, providing information about their potential as therapeutics for a range of medical diseases. Herbs such as echinacea, elderberry, and astragalus, for example, have been investigated for their immunomodulatory qualities; some studies have shown promise in lowering the intensity and length of respiratory infections. In a similar vein, plants with anti-inflammatory properties, including devil's claw, Boswellia, and turmeric, have attracted interest and shown potential to reduce symptoms related to diseases like rheumatoid arthritis and osteoarthritis. Additionally, the anxiolytic and sedative qualities of plants, including valerian, passionflower, and kava, have been studied, providing alternate possibilities for treating anxiety and sleep disturbances.

Clinical trials and observational studies are essential for clarifying the safety profile of herbal therapies in addition to assessing efficacy. Contrary to popular belief, herbal remedies can interact with prescription medications and pose risks, particularly to vulnerable populations. Researchers can minimize possible hazards and optimize health outcomes by providing evidence-based guidance for the safe and effective use of herbal remedies through systematic monitoring of adverse events and interactions. In addition, combining traditional knowledge with modern evidence, advancing cultural competence, and maintaining indigenous healing methods depend on the cooperation of traditional healers, community members, and scientific researchers.

The assessment of the effectiveness of herbal interventions still needs to overcome a number of obstacles despite the advancements in the field of herbal medicine research. Creating solid evidence that can survive scrutiny and guide therapeutic practice is hampered by a lack of funding, biases in study designs, and non-standard processes. Furthermore, there are disparities in quality control, labeling, and marketing strategies because of the vast variations in regulatory frameworks that apply to herbal products across different jurisdictions. In order to address these issues, legislators, scientists, and medical professionals must work together to advance scientific integrity, accountability, and openness in the field of herbal medicine research.

To sum up, observational research and clinical trials are essential resources for assessing the safety and effectiveness of herbal therapies. Researchers can produce thorough evidence to support public health efforts, policy recommendations, and healthcare decisions by combining the advantages of both approaches. In addition, cultivating interdisciplinary partnerships and using culturally aware methodologies are critical to closing the knowledge gap between conventional wisdom and contemporary research, encouraging reciprocity, and advancing fair access to herbal therapies across the globe. Realizing the full potential of herbal medicine to enhance health and well- being will require embracing evidence-based procedures and encouraging communication amongst varied stakeholders as the field develops.

CONCLUSION

In "Phytomedicines to Combat Viruses. In his work "Harnessing the Power of Botanicals in Viral Infections," the author carefully examines how botanical treatments may be used to treat viral infections. A gripping story that highlights the rich heritage and many uses of herbal medicine throughout cultures and civilizations is told throughout the book. The publication delves into a multitude of information, highlighting the significant influence of botanicals on viral infections while also navigating through traditional traditions and contemporary scientific developments.

The book's impressive accomplishment is its integration of conventional knowledge with recent research. The author offers a comprehensive viral treatment and prevention strategy by combining cutting-edge scientific discoveries with ancient healing traditions. This combination of traditional knowledge and contemporary research advances both our knowledge of herbal medicine and opens new avenues for therapeutic application.

Additionally, "Herbal Strategies Against Viruses" provides helpful advice on recognizing, preparing, and using herbal treatments. Readers are equipped to take advantage of the therapeutic potential of botanicals in their own lives with the help of thorough explanations and recommendations based on solid data. For those looking for natural solutions for managing viruses, the book offers thorough guidance on everything from growing medicinal plants to making herbal remedies.

The article also emphasizes the value of cooperation between scientists, healthcare professionals, and traditional healers. The book promotes a synergistic approach to viral healthcare by encouraging interdisciplinary collaboration and conversation. This approach combines the best aspects of herbal therapy with conventional medicine in a harmonious manner.

Ultimately, "Herbal Strategies Against Viruses" proves to be a ground-breaking tool that cuts over disciplinary lines and sheds light on the medicinal plants' capacity to heal viral diseases. In the never-ending search for efficient viral management, the book's richness of information, helpful advice, and integrated viewpoint serve as a light of empowerment.

Thank you for buying and reading/ listening to our book. If you found this book useful/ helpful please take a few minutes and leave a review on the platform where you purchased our book. Your feedback matters greatly to us.

9 798869 311788